Foundations of Psychiatric Mental Health Nursing

Foundations of Psychiatric Mental Health Nursing

As per INC Syllabus

Shija K Msc (N) MA (Public Admin.)
Assistant Professor
Government College of Nursing
Thiruvananthapuram, India

Jija D Msc (N) PhD
Assistant Professor
Government College of Nursing
Thiruvananthapuram, India

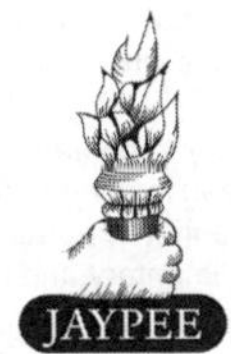

JAYPEE BROTHERS MEDICAL PUBLISHERS
The Health Sciences Publisher
New Delhi | London

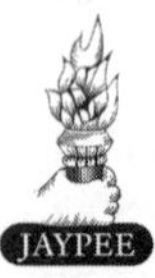

Jaypee Brothers Medical Publishers (P) Ltd

Headquarters
EMCA House
23/23-B, Ansari Road, Daryaganj
New Delhi - 110 002, India
Landline: +91-11-23272143, +91-11-23272703
+91-11-23282021, +91-11-23245672
E-mail: jaypee@jaypeebrothers.com

Corporate Office
4838/24, Ansari Road, Daryaganj
New Delhi - 110 002, India
Phone: +91-11-43574357
Fax: +91-11-43574314
E-mail: jaypee@jaypeebrothers.com

Overseas Office
J.P. Medical Ltd
83 Victoria Street, London
SW1H 0HW (UK)
Phone: +44 20 3170 8910
E-mail: info@jpmedpub.com

EU GPSR Authorised Representative
Logos Europe, 9 rue Nicolas Poussin
17000, La Rochelle, France
Phone: +33 (0) 6 67 93 73 78
E-mail: contact@logoseurope.eu

Website: www.jaypeebrothers.com
Website: www.jaypeedigital.com

Inquiries for bulk sales may be solicited at: jaypee@jaypeebrothers.com

Foundations of Psychiatric Mental Health Nursing

First Edition: **2018, Reprint: 2026**

ISBN: 978-93-5270-183-4

Printed at: Samrat Offset Pvt. Ltd.

Dedicated

To

Our Students

Preface

Foundations of Psychiatric Mental Health Nursing has been written with the aim of providing knowledge on psychiatric nursing based on the INC syllabus specified for the diploma nursing students. However, it will be useful for the graduate nursing students as well as for the nurses who practice in psychiatric clinical setting.

Each chapter is written in short and comprehensible language in order to facilitate the learning process based on nursing process approach and specified the role of nurse in every sphere of care.

Organization of the Textbook

This textbook has been organised into 17 chapters.

- Chapter 1 deals with the concept of mental health and mental illness.
- Chapter 2 includes history and development of psychiatric nursing with emphasis on community health programmes.
- Chapters 3 and 4 deal with the communication, therapeutic nurse-patient relationship and the methods of assessing a patient with mental illness.
- Chapter 5 deals with the etiology and symptomatology of mental disorders.
- Chapter 6 covers the different therapeutic modalities used in psychiatry with due emphasis on the role of nurse in these therapies.
- Chapters 7 to 14 deal with the definition, etiology, clinical features, treatment and nursing management of clients with different psychiatric disorders based on nursing process approach.
- Chapter 15 covers the concept of community mental health, prevention of mental disorders and the role of nurse in community mental health services.
- Chapter 16 deals with the management of psychiatric emergencies and the role of nurse in crisis intervention.
- Chapter 17 discusses the legal aspects in psychiatry and specifies the legal responsibilities of nurse. The Mental Health Act, 2017 has been incorporated into this chapter.

This book is intended to equip the students to have an overview of various aspects related to psychiatric nursing and provide quality care to the mentally ill based on the principles of psychiatric nursing.

Shija K
Jija D

Acknowledgments

We would like to express our sincere gratitude to M/s Jaypee Brothers Medical Publishers for their inappreciable effort in making this textbook a reality.

We are also extremely thankful to all the teachers who instilled knowledge throughout our educational path.

Ms Jincy Ann Paul and Ms Athira VS deserve special mention for their help during this endeavor.

We also place on the record the extensive help and encouragement provided by our parents and all our family members.

INC Syllabus

MENTAL HEALTH NURSING

Placement: Second Year **Time: 70 hours**

Course Description:

This course is designed to help students to develop the concept of mental health and mental illness, its causes, symptoms, prevention, treatment, modalities and nursing management of mentally ill for individual, family and community.

General Objective

Upon completion of this course, the students shall able to:

- Describe the concept of mental health and mental illness and the emerging trends in psychiatric nursing.
- Explain the causes and factors of mental illness, its prevention and control.
- Identify the symptoms and dynamic of abnormal human behavior in comparison with normal human behavior.
- Demonstration of a desirable attitude and skills in rendering comprehensive nursing care to the mentally ill.

Unit	*Learning Objectives*	*Content*	*Hour*	*Learning Activites*	*Methods of Assess-ment*	*Chapter*
I	Describe the concept of mental health and mental illness in relation to providing comprehen-sive care to the patients	**Introduction** • Concept of mental health and mental Illness • Misconceptions related to mental illness • Principles of Mental health nursing • Definition of terms used in psychiatry • Review of defense mechanisms • Mental Health Team	5	Lecture cum dis-cussions Struc-tured discussion Group interac-tion	Short answers Objective type	1

Unit	*Learning Objectives*	*Content*	*Hour*	*Learning Activites*	*Methods of Assessment*	*Chapter*
II	Narrate the historical development of Psychiatry and psychiatric nursing	**History of Psychiatry** • History of Psychiatric Nursing - India and at international level • Trends in Psychiatric Nursing • National mental health programme	4	Lecture cum discussions	Short answers Objective type	2
III	Describe mental health assessment	**Mental Health Assessment** • Psychiatry history taking • Mental status examination • Interview technique	4	Lecture cum discussions Demonstration	Short answers Objective type Return demonstration	4
IV	Describe therapeutic relationship Demonstrate skills in process recording	**Therapeutic nurse-patient relationship:** • Therapeutic nurse-patient relationship: Definition, components and phases, Importance • Communication skills. Definition, elements, types, factors influencing communication, barriers (therapeutic impasse)	5	Lecture cum discussions Role play Videos Demonstration of process recording	Short answers Return demonstration	3
V	List various mental disorders and describe their mental and psychiatric and nursing management	**Mental Disorders and Nursing Interventions** • Psycho-Pathophysiology of human behavior • Etiological theories (genetics, biochemical, psychological, etc) • Classification of mental disorders	25	Lecture cum discussions Case study Case presentation Process recording	Short answers Essay types Case study Case presentation	5

Unit	*Learning Objectives*	*Content*	*Hour*	*Learning Activites*	*Methods of Assessment*	*Chapter*
		• Disorders of thought, motor activity, perception, mood, speech, memory, concentration, judgment • Prevalence, etiology, signs and symptoms, prognosis, medical and nursing management		Videos Role plays Field visits- De-addiction centers, Alcohol Anonyms group, Adolescent clinics, Child guidance centers, etc.		
		• Personality and types of personality related to psychiatric disorder				12
		• Organic mental disorders: Delirium, Dementia				7
		• Psychotic disorders: - Schizophrenic disorders				9
		- Mood (affective) disorders: Mania depression, Bipolar affective disorders (BPAD)				10
		• Neurotic disorders: Phobia, anxiety disorders, obsessive compulsive disorders, depressive neurosis, conversion disorders, dissociative reaction, psychosomatic disorders, post traumatic stress disorder				11
		• Substance use and de-addiction: Alcohol, tobacco and other psychoactive substance				8

Unit	Learning Objectives	Content	Hour	Learning Activites	Methods of Assessment	Chapter
		• Child and adolescent psychiatric disorder: - Sleep disorder - Eating disorders - Sexual disorders • Nursing Management: Nursing process and process recording in caring for patients with various psychiatric disorders				14 13 7–14
VI	Describe the Bio – psychosocial therapies and explain the role of the nurse	**Bio–Psycho and Social Therapies** • Psychopharmacology–Definition, classification of drugs antipsychotic, Antidepressant, antimanic, antianxiety agents, anti parkinsons • Psychosocial therapies – individual therapies, group therapy, behavior therapy, occupational therapy, family therapy, melieu therapy • Role of nurse in these therapies • Somatic therapy–Electro Convulsive Therapy, insulin therapy • Role of nurse in these therapies	12	Lecture cum discussions Seminar Videos Demonstration Field visits-Rehabilitation center, Day care centers Role plays	Short answers Essay types Return demonstration Quiz Drug study	6
VII	Describe the concept of preventive community mental health services	**Community Mental Health** • Concept, importance, scope • Attitudes, Stigma and discrimination related to the mentally ill	5	Lecture cum discussions Role play Videos	Short answers Essay type Assignment	15

Unit	*Learning Objectives*	*Content*	*Hour*	*Learning Activites*	*Methods of Assessment*	*Chapter*
	Enumerate the nurse's role in National mental health programme	• Prevention of mental illness (Preventive Psychiatry) during childhood, adolescent, adulthood and old age • Community Mental Health Services • Role of Nurse in national mental health programme and Psychiatric care in Community				
VIII	Explain different psychiatric emergencies and their management Demonstrate skills in crisis intervention	**Psychiatric Emergencies and Crisis Intervention** • Types of Psychiatric emergencies: Over Active, under active patient, Violent behavior, • Suicide, adverse drug reactions, withdrawal symptoms, acute psychosis, etc • Crisis and its intervention: AIDS, Adolescent Crisis	5	Lecture cum discussions Videos Role plays Demonstration	Short answers Objective type Essay type	16
IX	Describe the legal aspects to be kept in mind in the care of mentally ill patients	**Forensic Psychiatry/ Legal Aspects** • India Lunatic Act 1912 • Narcotic Drugs and psychotropic Act 1965, 1985 • Mental Health Act 1987, 2014 • Admission and discharge procedures	5	Lecture cum discussions Demonstration	Short answers Essay type Objective quiz	17

Unit	*Learning Objectives*	*Content*	*Hour*	*Learning Activites*	*Methods of Assessment*	*Chapter*
		• Standards of psychiatric nursing practice • Rights of Mentally ill patients • Legal responsibilities in the care of mentally ill patients				Incorporated in chapter 1

Contents

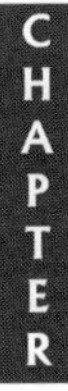

1 Introduction

The concepts of health, mental health and mental illness have evolved after many years of efforts by theorists/scientists and become more refined after discussions.

An overview of defense mechanisms will help in easy understanding of mental health and mental illness.

REVIEW OF DEFENSE MECHANISMS

Defense Mechanisms (Ego Defense)

These are the psychological means of coping with conflict or anxiety, that operates at an unconscious level, and help the individual to be away from unpleasant feelings or help to feel better.

Unpleasant or unacceptable memories, drives or wishes that are banished to the unconscious or subconscious mind do not disappear. They continue to exert a powerful influence on behavior. The forces, which try to keep painful or socially undesirable thoughts and memories out of the conscious mind, are termed defense mechanisms.

Defense mechanisms are used to protect ourselves from feelings of anxiety or guilt, which make us feel threatened. As id or superego are very much demanding, conflicts arise. But these are not under one's conscious control. With the ego, one involuntarily use one or more mental mechanisms to protect self from stressful situations in life. Ego-defense mechanisms are natural and normal.

When the ego defenses become out of proportion, or inappropriate, neuroses such as anxiety states, phobias, obsessions, or hysteria occur. Maladaptive use of defense mechanisms promotes disintegration of ego and will lead to loss of ability to deal with reality, with interpersonal relations and with occupational functioning.

Types

There are many mental mechanisms that are commonly used in everyday life. They are:

Compensation

Consciously covering one's own weakness by giving more emphasize on it or by making up this weakness by focusing on a desirable trait that is already existing.

Example: A student who is weak in mathematics will overwork on mathematics to compensate for the weakness. or

A student who is weak in academic performance will compensate by focusing on arts/sports which he likes, feels more comfortable.

Displacement

Displacement is the redirection of an impulse (usually aggression) from the real target to a less powerful substitute target. The target can be a person or an object that can be a symbolic one.

Example: Someone who gets shouting from the superior may go home and kick the pet or shout at or beat up a family member.

Denial

Denial is the blocking of existence of real events and its associated feelings from awareness as if they are unreal. Individual unconsciously refuses to admit an unacceptable event or refuses to face the difficult situation. He will try to avoid the stressful situation by denying it.

Example: Alcoholics may refuse to admit to themselves that it is bad for their health.

Substitution

It is the mechanism in which unattainable goals are replaced with an attainable goal and thus frustrations are avoided.

Example: A student who desires to be a doctor, but not qualified in medical entrance will substitute it with nursing.

Identification

Individual's effort to increase self-worth by acquiring or imitating the characteristics of someone else who is a famous or hero. Seen during adolescence by identifying themselves with film actors or actress. This helps the child further develop the adult ego state and the parent ego state.

Example: After joining in student police cadet, a student decide to become a police by identifying himself with the police officers.

Introjection

Characteristics of significant person (attitudes, messages, prejudices) are subconsciously integrates to self and separation of it from self is difficult. It is the internalization of another person's believes and values.

Example: After joining nursing, the student integrates herself with the senior staff nurse who won a national award for service.

Reaction Formation

The person behaves by showing exaggerated form of opposite feelings and behavior for preventing the expression of real unacceptable thoughts.

Example: The student who does not like a very strict teacher may display himself or herself as over polite and very much loving.

Sublimation

It is a mental mechanism with which unacceptable emotions and drives are displaced in a socially acceptable manner, rather than in destructive. It is the healthy redirection of an emotion.

Example: Instead of acting out of anger on your friends, the boy may go to the gym for physical workout.

Repression

This is the most important and first defense mechanism that Freud discovered. Repression is an unconscious mechanism employed by the ego to keep disturbing, unpleasant threatening thoughts from becoming conscious, or it is unconscious forgetting.

Repression is the involuntary or unconscious blocking of painful or unpleasant thoughts and memories out of awareness and forgetting them.

This is not a very successful defense in long-term as it pushes the wishes, ideas or memories into the unconscious mind.

Example: A person with history of physical abuse in childhood may forget about it and will be unable to memorize it as he/she grows.

Suppression

Suppression is the voluntary blocking of distressing thoughts or feelings from one's awareness. But it can be memorized as it is pushed to the subconscious mind.

Example: A girl voluntarily blocks the memories of witnessing an accident.

Regression

This is an unconscious return to the childish or primitive psychological time when one is in stress. When we are frightened, our behaviors often become more childish or primitive. A child when faces a change or stress he/she may begin to restart thumb sucking or bedwetting.

Example: A girl starts bedwetting after the arrival of her father from military, who is strict in dealings.

Rationalization

Rationalization is the cognitive distortion of 'the facts' to justify unacceptable feelings. Individual justifies his failures and socially unacceptable behavior by giving socially approved reasons.

This may take two forms as sour grape mechanism and sweet lemon mechanism.

In sour grape mechanism, individual himself blames the unattainable task or things by showing its negative side of it as in case of wolf and the grapes story. It is an intellectual way to diminish pain or guilt.

In sweet lemon mechanism, the individual justifies his status or limitations by highlighting the advantages of what he has.

Projection

Individuals attribute their unacceptable thoughts, feeling and motives to another person, or they are projected to others and thus seeks relief from anxiety. Unconsciously or consciously individual blames others for one's own problems.

Example: Aggressive thoughts, sexual fantasies, etc. may be attributed to others.

Blaming the teacher for the failure in exam.

Isolation

Here memory or thoughts are separated from emotions related to it. Individual can remember and talk about a traumatic experience without feeling any emotion. The person talks about the incident as a third person's perception, or as a happening to another person.

Example: A person who is kidnapped by terrorist explains about his sufferings, without any emotional response.

Intellectualization

Avoidance of emotions of a painful event by using intellectual process. Individual realizes/acknowledges the facts, but not the emotions related to that.

Example: Individual will not show any emotions while describing the accident and death of his father by realizing the underlying mistake or problem.

Undoing

Doing something consciously to make up for a wrong doing that had occurred previously.

Example: Taking the child for an outing after beating him or punishing.

Conversion

It is the defense mechanism by which mental conflict or anxiety is converted to a physical symptom as paralysis, blindness without any medical basis. This anxiety is usually arousing from repressed feelings or wishes.

Example: A soldier on being deployed into battle is conflicted about his desire to serve country but believes it is wrong to kill for any reason develops paralysis, blindness, or deafness with no medical cause.

Dissociation

Unconscious separation of painful feelings/emotions from unacceptable idea, situation or object.

DEFINITION OF TERMS USED IN PSYCHIATRY

- **Mind:** Mind is a set of neurocognitive functions including consciousness perception, thinking, judgment and memory that keeps one alert and oriented. There is no globally accepted definition for mind.
- **Psychiatry:** It is the branch of medicine that deals with the diagnosis, treatment and prevention of mental illness.
- **Psychiatrist:** Medical doctor with special training in psychiatry—as diploma/PG in psychiatry, accountable for diagnosis and treatment of mentally ill.
- **Stress:** A state of disequilibrium resulting from a disharmony between demands occurring within environment of the individual (internal/external) and his/her coping ability with that demands (Townsend M).
- **Crisis:** Psychological disequilibrium resulting from hazardous circumstances that constitute important problems that are difficult for the individual to solve or to escape from (Townsend M).
- **Adjustment:** It is the behavioral process of balancing conflicting needs or needs against obstacles in the environment (Encyclopaedia Britannica).

  A series of adjustments begin when there is a need and they ends when the need is satisfied.
- **Adaptation:** It is the ability to adjust to new information and experiences or it is the restoration to homeostasis or equilibrium following a stress.
- **Eustress:** Positive and motivating stress, where individual shows ability to master a challenge or a stressor.

- **Behavior:** It is the sum total of all activities of a human being, with cognitive, affective and psychomotor elements.
- **Psychopathology:** It is the scientific study of mental disorders that include etiology, classification, manifestations and treatment.
- **Abnormal behavior:** Deviation of covert and overt activities of a person from normal behavior as per the social norms.
  There are 4D's which define abnormality.
  1. **Distress:** It is the negative feelings by the individual as deeply troubled and affected by their illness.
  2. **Dysfunction:** It is the maladaptive behavior in individual's ability to perform normal daily functions.
  3. **Deviance:** Specific thoughts, behaviors and emotions that are unacceptable and unusual in a society or culture is considered as deviance.
  4. **Danger:** Dangerous or violent behavior directed to individual himself or to others in the environment (homicidal and suicidal activities).
- **Mental illness:** Maladaptive responses to stressors evidenced by thoughts, feelings and behaviors that are not appropriate to the social norms and interferes with one's social, occupational and physical functioning (Townsend M).
- **Insanity:** It is a term that indicates that the individual is incompetent to manage his affairs and unable to foresee the effect of his action.
- **Maladaptation:** A failure of the body to regain homeostasis, following stress responses that are physiological and/or psychological, and disrupts the personal integrity of the individual. Maladaptation is an adaptation that is less helpful than harmful (Townsend M).
- **Personality:** Deeply ingrained patterns of behavior, which include the way one related to, perceives and thinks about the environment and oneself (Townsend M).
- **Psychosis:** A mental state in which there is loss of contact with reality and symptoms as delusions, hallucinations, disorganized speech patterns and bizarre or catatonic behavior (Townsend M).
- **Neurosis:** An unconscious conflict that produces anxiety, and other symptoms and leads to maladaptive use of defense mechanisms (Townsend M).
- **Psychotic disorder:** A serious psychiatric disorder in which there is a gross disorganization of the personality, marked disturbance in reality testing, impairments in interpersonal functioning and relationship to the external world (Townsend M).
- **Neurotic disorder:** Less serious psychiatric disorder characterized by excessive anxiety and/or depression, disrupted bodily functions, unsatisfying interpersonal relationship, and behaviors that interferes

with routine functioning. There is no loss of touch with the reality (Townsend M).

- **Disaster:** A natural or man made occurrence that overwhelms the resources of an individual or community and increased the need for emergency evacuation and medical services (Townsend M).

CONCEPT OF MENTAL HEALTH AND MENTAL ILLNESS

Introduction

The concept of health had become more refined with long-term efforts at international level. World Health Organisation (WHO) defines health as 'a state of complete physical, mental and social well-being and not merely the absence of disease or infirmity'. This definition itself shows that there is no health without mental health. Body-mind relationship shows that physical and mental health is interrelated. Mental health being the invisible part of health, people are not giving the due concern for it. But in the present scenario, the relevance of mental health is increasing because poor mental health is the basis for most of the social problems. Mental health is essential for the well-being of individual, family, society and thus that of nation.

Mental Health

Mental health is not merely the absence of major mental illness like schizophrenia or mood disorders and/or minor mental disorders like anxiety disorders or obsessive compulsive disorders. It is the ability to adapt to the changes and challenges in personal and social life and thus to maintain a state of harmony between self and others. Personality development, intelligence, attitude, habits and support systems contribute to one's mental health.

Definitions

- Mental health is 'simultaneous success at working, loving and creating with the capacity for mature and flexible resolutions of conflicts between instincts, conscience, other important people, and reality'. (**American Psychiatric Association —APA, 1980**)
- Mental health is a state of well-being in which an individual realizes his or her own abilities, can cope with the normal stresses of life, can work productively and is able to make a contribution to his or her community. **(WHO 2001)**
- Mental health is the state of simultaneous success at establishing and sustaining harmonious relationship with others by realizing one's own strength and weakness, by managing stress effectively and by working productively for the society.

Indicators of Mental Health

Many theorists have attempted to define/conceptualize mental health. Jahoda (1958) had pointed out six major indicators of mental health, and got wide acceptance.

1. **Positive attitude towards self**: The individual who has strong sense of personal worth and identity will feel secure in his environment. Real perception of self (awareness and acceptance of strength and weakness of self) will help one to have positive outlook.
2. **Growth, development and the ability for self-actualization:** The individual successfully achieves the definite tasks with each developmental stage, and thus gains motivation to his or her highest potentials.
3. **Integration:** This involves the person's ability for successful adaptation to the environment and ability for development of own philosophy of life. This will help him/her to keep anxiety at manageable levels during stressful situations. All these contribute to a balance among various life process.
4. **Autonomy:** It is the individual's ability to make own choices and to accept responsibilities for the outcome. This will enable one to perform tasks in an independent and self-directed manner.
5. **Perception of reality:** It is the real perception of the environment without distortions and necessitates respect and concern for the needs and wants of others. Or empathy and social sensitivity are of special concern here.
6. **Environmental mastery:** It is the ability of individual to achieve satisfactory role within the group, society or environment. The individual is able to love others and to accept the love of others. Individual will be able to strategize, make decisions, change, adjust and adapt to the environment and thus mastery give satisfaction.

Factors Affecting Mental Health

- **Genetic factors:** Mental health as well as mental illness are seems to be inherited. Studies have proven that mental illness is more in some families or it runs in families. In such families mental health will be poor.
- **Physiological factors:** Mental health is influenced by the hormonal changes in our body during different developmental stages and endocrine disorders, e.g. puberty, pregnancy and puerperium, menopause, and disorders like hypo/hyperthyroidism.
- **Physical ill health:** Physical illness, disabilities, and injuries also may affect one's mental health.
- **Psychological factors:** Good parenting, happy childhood, good family relationships, schooling and social relations can contribute

to good mental health, which is indicated by self-esteem or positive self-image, feeling of being loved, accepted and self-confidence. Maternal deprivation, and deprivation of physical and emotional care, abuse/trauma in childhood are some factors that can negatively affect mental health. Abuse—physical, sexual, psychological or verbal can lead to poor mental health and sometimes can lead to mental illness in future.

- **Social factors/environmental factors:** Good socioeconomic status, social norms, healthy living conditions, healthy lifestyle, mutually respecting cultural attitude and relations can add mental health.
  Poor socioeconomic background, unhealthy living conditions, strained relationships, slum areas, strict social rules—all these can negatively affect mental health.

For the maintenance of good mental health, good interpersonal relations, effective use of defense mechanism and good support system (family, society, friends and service from other resources) are essential.

Characteristics of Mentally Healthy Individual

A mentally healthy individual is with the following features:

- High self-esteem, self-discipline and self-confidence.
- Altruistic and has capacity for intimacy.
- Social competence and maintains satisfying relationship.
- Respects and love themselves and others.
- Resilience: It is the ability to bounce back from adversity.
- Control over their emotions: They are not overwhelmed by emotions like anger, fear, love, happiness.
- Autonomy: They will be independent in all their decisions and activities.
- Environmental mastery: They have a sense of control over their lives and meets challenges and solve problems. They are able to accept disappointments also. They have their own philosophy of life.
- Desire for self-actualization: They take reasonable risk to grow and also balance with work, rest and recreation.
- Creativity: They are creative and appreciates the creativeness of others.
- Emotional intelligence: Emotional intelligence is the ability to identify and mange your own emotions and the emotions of others.

Mental Illness

Due to the changes in cultural factors, a universal concept of mental illness is difficult. Mental illness is indicated by abnormal behavior. But the concepts of normal and abnormal behavior are difficult to find out, because they are influenced by and varied with sociocultural factors.

Definitions

APA in its DSM V classification defines mental disorders as—A syndrome characterized by clinically significant disturbances in a individual's cognitions, emotions, regulations or behavior that reflects a dysfunctions in the psychological, biological and developmental process underlying mental functions (APA 2013).

Mental and behavioral disorders are understood as clinically significant conditions characterized by alterations in thinking, mood (emotions) or behavior associated with personal distress and/or impaired functioning (WHO 2001).

Mental disorders are syndromes characterized by disturbance in one's thoughts, perception, cognition, emotions and behaviors that are not culturally appropriate.

Characteristics of Mental Illness

- Mental illness is characterized by maladjustment in usual life situations and thus causes disharmony in individual's ability to do self-care in an effective manner.
- Change in thinking, perception, emotions, memory, judgment and insight results in changes in speech and behavior, which are not matching with one's previous personality and also with the norms of society.
- The behavior changes result in sufferings or distress to the individual, others or both, thus will affect the activities of daily living and relationship with others.
- Changes in activities further add the distress and leads to social and vocational dysfunction (disturbances in daily activities, work and relationship with important others).

Characteristics of mentally ill person: Some characteristic features of mental illness are listed. But all these features will not coexist in single patient.

- Deviation from social norms.
- Biological dysfunctions (change in sleep, appetite, sexual desire, and activity level)
- Maladaptive/bizarre behavior
- Inappropriate emotions
- Abnormal perceptions
- Inability to resolve conflicts
- Self-destructive behavior
- Lack of insight or impaired insight
- Disturbance in thought process
- Irrational beliefs

- Lack of real perceptions of environment
- Impaired cognitive functions
- Poor interpersonal relationships
- Constant anxiety and fear
- Poor impulse control
- Ritualistic behavior
- Difficulty with adaptation
- Dependence on chemicals.

MISCONCEPTIONS RELATED TO MENTAL ILLNESS

There are many misconceptions about mental disorders, that divert people from treating it as an illness. These myths make the early detection and treatment more difficult.

Common myths about mental illness in India are as follows:

- **Mental illness is the result of evil spirit or black magic:** Even now people are consulting astrologists and attends prayer sessions in treating mental illness.
  - *Fact:* Mental illness usually occur due to biopsychosocial factors and this can only be treated with drugs and psychosocial therapies. Prayer and religiosity can increase their confidence and optimism.
- **Psychiatric disorder means a single disease and reflects personal weakness or personality flaw.**
  - *Fact:* Mental disorders indicate a group of illness that vary in nature. Neurotransmitters or the chemical messengers are responsible for normal mental functioning. An imbalance of these chemicals lead to serious mental illness. Persistent stressors can also lead to mental illness. Personal weakness itself is not the single responsible factor.
- **Mental disorders are hereditary:**
  - *Fact:* Hereditary factors when combined with psychological and social factors, it can lead to mental illness. Like any physical illness, there is some genetic background for mental illness also.
- **Mental disorders affect very few people or prevalence of mental illness is low:**
  - *Fact:* Mental illness is common. It affects people of all ages, gender, education and culture.
- **Abnormal behavior is bizarre and mentally ill are dangerous and violent:**
  - *Fact:* Mentally ill persons show maladaptive behavior. Most of them don't show bizarre/dangerous behavior.

- **Normal person can never be abnormal:**
  - *Fact:* Behavior is said to be normal or abnormal by considering the social norms. A person cannot remain normal all the time. Anybody can become abnormal at any time due to biopsychosocial factors.
- **Patients admitted to mental hospital are more problematic than those in general hospitals:**
  - *Fact:* Whether the person is admitted in mental hospital or general hospital, they will be treated by psychiatrists, and like physical illness, mental illness also has effective treatment.
- **Mental health and physical health are not related to each other:**
  - *Fact:* Body and mind are interrelated. Mentally ill people have its effect in physical health and people who suffer from physical illness may experience mental health problems like anxiety or depression.
- **Once mentally ill, it will persist in the entire life:**
  - *Fact:* Mental illness can be effectively treated with drugs and psychosocial therapies. Newer drugs are more effective and with less side effect.
- **Mentally ill need to be treated separately—in mental hospitals:**
  - *Fact:* Now there is mental health services at District hospitals, and at PHC/CHC's via District Mental Health Programme clinics. Many of them are treated on outpatient basis.
- **Mental illness is something to be ashamed of**:
  - *Fact:* There is nothing to be ashamed for seeking treatment from mental health center. Like physical illness, mental illness also can occur at any time and can be treated. Do not hesitate in treating any illness.
- **Mental illness can be treated with marriage:**
  - *Fact:* Marriage is not a treatment for mental illness. Marriage usually increases the risk for relapse.
- **Mental illness will not affect children:**
  - *Fact:* Mental illness can occur at any age.

MENTAL HEALTH NURSING

Due to rapid urbanization, social, economic, demographic and technological changes, mental health and behavioral problems are increasing and it imposes many challenges worldwide.

In India also substance abuse, and other psychiatric disorders are increasing. This increases the scope and relevance of Mental Health and Psychiatric Nursing. Mental health nursing has application in other specialties of nursing, because psychological aspects of care is vital in developmental stages, crises and in any illness—physical or mental.

Definitions

Psychiatric nursing is a specialized area of nursing practice, employing the wide range of explanatory theories of human behavior as its science and purposeful use of self as its art (American Nurses Association, 2000).

Psychiatric nursing focuses on the care and rehabilitation of people with identifiable mental illness or disorders.

Mental Health Nursing aims the prevention of mental illness by focusing on well and at risk population or to provide immediate treatment for those with early signs of disorders.

Psychiatric-mental health nursing is the diagnosis and treatment of human response to actual or potential mental health problems (ANA and International Society of Psychiatric-Mental Health Nurses, 2000).

In Mental health and Psychiatric Nursing, care may be focused at an individual, family, group, organizations or community or specific population (elderly, women, children, adolescents, youth, mentally challenged and people with chronic mental illness).

Principles of Mental Health Nursing

In mental health nursing some basic principles should be followed:

1. **Patient is accepted exactly as he is:** Acceptance conveys a feeling of being loved and cared. Acceptance does not mean complete permissiveness, but setting of positive behavior to convey respect as an individual human being. Nurse should convey that she may not approve everything; and he will not be judged or rejected because of his behavior.

Acceptance can be expressed in the following ways:

- **Being non-judgmental and non-punitive:** Patient's behavior should not be judged as right or wrong, good or bad, and should not be punished for his/her undesirable behavior. Any sort of punishment (direct punishment like chaining/restraining, keeping in separate room) and indirect punishment as ignoring the presence, withdrawing attentions, etc.) should be avoided.
- **Show interest in the patient as a person:** Sincere interest to the Patient can be shown by:
  - Observing and studying the patient behavior pattern.
  - Being aware of patient's like and dislikes.
  - Permitting him to make his choices and decisions.
  - Be honest and avoid false reassurance.
  - If any demand cannot be met, explain the reason.
  - Deal his comments, complaints and expressions in realistic manner.
  - Spend time with patient and listen to him with interest.
  - Accept his fears as real to him.
  - Avoid sensitive topics and issues.

- **Recognize and reflect on feelings which the patient may express:** Nurse should have the skill to identify the actual feeling which is expressed, while they talk. Both the content of speech and the expressed feelings underlying that will be recognised and reflected. **Example:** 'I am a dead person'—it means he feels worthless.
- **Talk with a purpose:** Nurses' interaction with the patient must revolve around patient's needs, wants and interests. Nurses' talk or responses must guide the patient. Use of understanding responses and avoidance of hostile, evaluating and probing questions can help the patient to explore his feelings.
- **Listening:** Nurse should actively listen to what the patient says and allow him/her to express the strongly held feeling. Both verbal and non-verbal responses should be considered.
- **Permit the expression of strongly held feelings:** Allow the patient to express strong feelings without disapproval or punishment. Accept strong negative feelings (anxiety, fear, hostility) quietly and calmly.

2. **Use self-understanding as a therapeutic tool:** Awareness of one's own feelings, attitudes and responses will help a psychiatric nurse to understand others. Nurses can understand themselves by:
   - Exchanging personal experience with colleagues.
   - Discussing our personal reactions with an experienced person.
   - Participating in group conferences relatives to patient care.
   - Introspecting why he/she feel, act and did.
3. **Consistency is used to contribute to patients' security:**
   - Consistency must be reflected in our attitudes, ward routine, and in setting limitations in patients.
   - Consistency should be maintained from nurse to nurse and shift to shift by definite planning (e.g. consistency in routine, health teaching, limit setting).
4. **Reassurance should be given in suitable and acceptable manner:** Reassurance builds patient's confidence or help to restore it. But do not make false promises.
   - Be truly interested in patient's problems.
   - Pay attention to patient's matters, even if they are not much significant.
   - Nurse has to analyze and understand the situation according to patient's level. Try to meet his/her needs without his/her demands and appreciate improvement.
   - Agree that patient has problems and think together to solve this and accept outlet of anxiety in him/her.
5. **Patients' behavior is changed through emotional experience and not by rational interpretations:** Major focus in psychiatry is

on the feeling aspect and not on the intellectual aspect. Advising or explaining is not effective in changing behavior. Corrective emotional experience given through psychodrama or role play can help the patient to gain insight about his behavior and may leads to desired behavior.

6. **Unnecessary increase in patient's anxiety should be avoided:** Factors that cause/increase anxiety in a patient will vary from individual to individual. But in general, nurses can avoid:
   - Showing attention or highlighting patient's deficits/failures.
   - Showing nurse's own anxiety.
   - Allowing patient to face repeated failures.
   - Putting difficult tasks/demands that cannot be fulfilled by patient.
   - Direct contradictions of patient's psychotic ideas.
   - Use of professional terms and sharp comments to the patient.
7. **Objective observation of patient helps to understand his behavior:** Objectivity is the ability to evaluate exactly what the patient wants to say, by not mixing it with one's own feeling, opinion or judgment. For this nurse should introspect and be sure that her own emotional needs are not influencing patient's needs.
8. **Maintain realistic nurse-patient relationship:** Realistic and professional relationship focuses on personal and emotional needs of patients, and not on nurse's needs. Nurse should be able to empathize and understand the feelings and behavior of patients.
9. **Avoid physical and verbal force as much as possible:** Nurse should be able to predict the patient's behavior, so that undesirable behavior can be prevented. Any sort of punishment should be avoided. Anger, annoyance, non-verbal comments must be avoided.
10. **Nursing care is centered on the patient as a person and not on the control of symptoms:** Nursing care should be focused on person's need, not on symptoms—because patients with same symptoms may have different needs. At the same time symptoms should be analyzed for understanding its meanings.
11. **Explanation of procedures and routines should be according to the level of understanding of the patient:** While giving explanations, consider the patients' level of anxiety, understanding and decision making ability. Explanations should not be withheld by thinking that patient has no touch with reality.
12. **Many procedures are modified, but basic principles remain unaltered:** Based on patient's needs, methods can be adapted, but underlying principles should remain the same.

Standards of Mental Health Nursing

In order to provide quality nursing care and to fulfill the profession's obligations, it is essential to have certain standards and these have to be maintained.

Standards of psychiatric nursing includes:

A. **Professional practice standards:**

- **Standard I—Theory:** Nurse applies scientifically sound and suitable theory as the basis for nursing practice.
- **Standard II—Assessment:** Nurse continuously do assessment and collects data in systematic, accurate and comprehensive manner. Data will be collected by behavioral observation, interviewing and physical and mental health assessment and sound judgments are made. A good rapport with the patient and family is essential for this. Assessment or data collection will lead to a conclusion and helps in further planning.
- **Standard III—Diagnosis:** Nursing diagnosis will be used as a basis for providing nursing care. Nurses provide care based on actual or potential problems that are within the scope of nursing. Collected data will be analyzed by comparing with norms, and finally identifies the problems with the patient and formulate nursing diagnoses and prioritize it.
- **Standard IV—Outcome identification:** Nurse's goal will be to influence the mental health outcome/to improve the patients' health status. So the expected outcome should be documented.
- **Standard V—Planning:** Nurses develop nursing care plan based on specific goals. This plan of care is used to guide interventions. Nurses identify appropriate nursing activities based on individual needs of each patient. Planning becomes more effective when it is done in collaboration with the patient, family and other members of mental health team.
- **Standard VI—Implementation/intervention:** Nurse implements the planned care for promotion and maintenance of physical and mental health and also for prevention of illness. Nurses can also focus on rehabilitation of the mentally ill.

  Intervention usually include psychoeducation, promotion of self-care activities, somatic therapies, providing therapeutic environment, counseling and psychotherapy. Nurse can also involve in community based services.
- **Standard VII—Evaluation:** Evaluation of the nursing care and patient's progress should be done in terms of the goal or expected outcome. Ongoing evaluation of the treatment and nursing care and modification of nursing process should be done. Needs of patients will vary from day-to-day and individual to individual.

B. **Standards of Professional Performance (American Nurses Association, 1991):**
   - **Standard I—Quality of care:** It can be done by evaluating the quality of nursing through peer review and performance appraisal.
   - **Standard II—Performance appraisal:** Nurse has to evaluate herself in terms of knowledge and practice and has to maintain the standards of performance. Performance can be appraised by the superior officers, and their feedback and suggestions also will be helpful in improvement of nursing care.
   - **Standard III—Education:** Nurses have to update their knowledge and skill through continuing education. Professional learning should be enhanced by attending conferences and workshops and has to be maintained throughout the service.
   - **Standard IV—Collegiality:** Psychiatric nurses have to share their knowledge, both theoretical and clinical practice, with the colleagues for the professional growth. Sharing knowledge, giving feedback and constructive criticism, motivation and support of colleagues will enable team work and mutual respect.
   - **Standard V—Ethics:** Psychiatric nurse has to maintain ethical consideration and standards in all her dealings with the patients and their caregivers because these patients are vulnerable population. We have to safeguard the patient's well-being and confidentiality is also important. Nurse needs to be thorough with the ethical code and should practice it as a legal/ethical responsibility.
   - **Standard VI—Collaboration:** Interdisciplinary collaboration with all health care professionals may contribute to effective planning, and decision making.
   - **Standard VII—Research:** Psychiatric nurses should participate in research activities—like conducting scientific studies, dissemination of findings and application of research findings in nursing practice.
   - **Standard VIII—Resource utilization:** Nurse should do patient advocacy on individual or group basis for utilizing cost effective resources and service. For this nurse should be a creative thinker and decision maker and must be aware of the political and economic status of that area.

Qualities of a Mental Health Nurse/Psychiatric Nurse

- **Awareness of self and acceptance of self:** Psychiatric nurse should have awareness of one's own feelings, professional and personal strengths and weakness and accepts them without feeling great or guilty. He/she should have his/her own philosophy of life.

- **Acceptance of the patient:** Nurse should accept the patient exactly as he is. It means unconditional acceptance as a person—not in terms of his behavior, color, socioeconomic class, etc.
- **Sincerity and interest in patient care:** This can be expressed by considering patient's interest, likes, problems and behavior. Nurse should show her interest in patient by listening and showing her concern to the clients and their families by instilling hope and at the same time by being honest. Nurse should try to anticipate and meet the needs of patients and their families, before they demand. These will help in adding their trust in nurse.
- **Empathy:** Empathy is the ability to keep yourself in other's position to experience their feelings and problems. Nurse must be able to imagine the feelings and experiences like hallucinations and delusion of patients, their distress and related problems in the family.
- **Reliability:** Nurse must be reliable person in all his/her duties and promises. Then only trusty relationship can be established.
- **Professionalism:** Maintain professionalism in all dealings with the patient and relatives.
- **Accountability:** Nurse should be accountable for quality care of life of patients.
- **Good knowledge and critical thinking:** Knowledge about abnormal behavior, different disorders, treatment, rehabilitation and nursing care along with critical thinking, problem-solving are essential. Theoretical knowledge should be correlated to clinical practice.

MENTAL HEALTH TEAM

Mental health team is a multidisciplinary team which is a collaboration of all professionals who belong to different discipline, and involved in the care of mentally ill. Interdisciplinary collaboration helps better coordination of their work in a complementary way. The final product of this will be a therapeutic environment.

The team members include mental health professionals like:

- **Psychiatrist:** It is a medical doctor who is specialized in mental health with postgraduation in Psychiatry. Their major responsibilities are diagnosis, medical care of mentally ill planning and deciding for other therapies. They take initiation in prevention of mental illness through their involvement in community based activities. He suggests other therapies and prescribes medication.
- **Clinical psychologist:** Needs to have doctoral degree in clinical psychology and should be a registered person. They perform diagnostic tests and involve in interpretation of findings of tests

and assessments. He/She can perform different psychosocial therapies. They can help the patients and their caregivers for better understanding, support and coping. They conduct counseling sessions to the patients and caregivers.

- **Psychiatric nurse:** A registered nurse with special training in psychiatric nursing. He/she has a central role in the care of psychiatric patients. She can work in both hospital and community settings. Nurses can provide both physical and psychological care to their patients, and must provide essential support and encouragement to the patient's families.
  - Nurse's responsibility include—daily care of patient, involvement in in-patient services, education of students, patients and their families, and community groups. The nurse can help the patient and family for better utilization of supportive services. She can conduct group therapies, counseling to individuals and family, and works as a part of organization. She can plan recreational sessions for the patients. Community psychiatric nurse can do follow-up after discharge from the hospitals.
- **Psychiatric social worker:** Psychiatric social worker should have a master degree in social work with special training in mental health settings. She/he will be accountable for community placement of patients and do the family case work, group therapy sessions and counseling also. They act as a liaison between the family, society and the hospital.

Psychiatric Paraprofessionals

- **Occupational therapists:** They are responsible for providing occupational training and other activity/programs related to it in the hospital settings. He/she should be a qualified occupational therapist and must have experience in mental health care settings. Based on the capacity and interest of patients, they are helped to gain skills, to gain an employment or to use leisure time creatively.
- **Counselor:** A person with qualification and experience in counseling can provide supportive counseling and psychoeducation if sufficient number of clinical psychologists are not available.
- **Recreational therapists/activity therapist:** Plans and engage the patients in some activities that stimulate them. This will help in improving interpersonal relationships, socialization and muscle coordination and thus more refined activities occur. This should be based on patient's interest and ability, otherwise it may increase their anxiety.
- **Play therapist:** Can do good observations and can provide good opportunities for play/recreation of children.

CONCLUSION

This chapter has dealt with the basics of mental health and mental health nursing. These concepts should always be there in mind when a mental health nurse deals with her patients in hospital or in community.

BIBLIOGRAPHY

1. Frisch N, Frisch L. Psychiatric Mental Health Nursing (Fourth Edition). Delmar Cengage Learning, New York, 2011.
2. Kapoor B. Textbook of Psychiatric Nursing. Delhi: Kumar Publishing House, 2014.
3. Lalitha K. Mental Health and Psychiatric Nursing. Delhi: CBS Publishers, 2009.
4. Sreevani R. A Guide to Mental Health and Psychiatric Nursing (Third Edition). New Delhi: Jaypee Brothers Medical Publishers (P) Ltd, 2016.
5. Stuart GW, Laraia MT. Principles and Practice of Psychiatric Nursing. St Louis: Mosby, 2001.
6. Townsend CM. Psychiatric Mental Health Nursing: Concepts of Care in Evidence-Based Practice (7th Edition). Philadelphia: FA Davis Company, 2012.

CHAPTER 2

History of Psychiatry

INTRODUCTION

Psychiatry is a branch of medicine which deals with the diagnosis, treatment and prevention of mental disorders. Mental illness existed very long back and it was always connected with superstitions and ignorance. History provides a way through which the past inspires the present and the present enriches the future.

HISTORY OF PSYCHIATRY: INTERNATIONAL

Hippocrates, father of medicine explained that mental disorders were caused by the imbalance of bodily humors. Temperaments were believed to be a mixture of 4 bodily humors—blood, phlegm, yellow bile and black bile.

History of psychiatry at the international level can be categorized into 5 periods such as:

1. **Period of persecution (1552 BC–1440 AD):** People believed that sound, black spirit or black magic causes mental illness. Insane were thrown out of the society and beaten up by the people. Treatment of mentally sick was based on the superstitious beliefs. Mentally ill were ill-treated and they had to take care of themselves.
2. **Period of segregation (1545 AD–1800 AD):** Middle Eastern Islamic countries believed that mental illness were caused by anger of God and witchcraft. Mentally ill were called insane and were placed in asylums. In 1547, Bethlehem hospital was constructed in London. Due to the pathetic condition that existed in that institution; it was corrected as Bedlam which means mad house.
3. **Humanitarian period (1745 AD–1826 AD):** Asylums were established and the physicians were more focused on moral treatment of mentally ill. Philippe Pinel insisted on humane and moral treatment of mentally ill. He removed

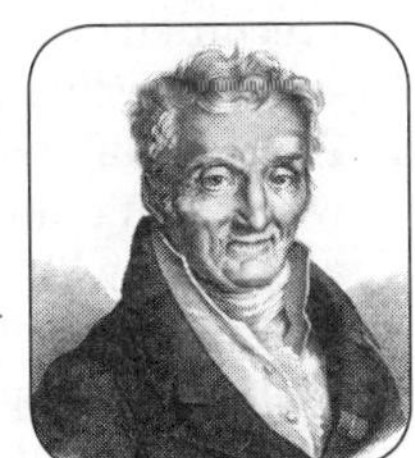
Philippe Pinel

chains of mentally ill. He was the Chief of Bicetre mental hospital and is referred as Father of modern psychiatry.

William Tuke in 1796 founded the York Retreat, where about 30 patients lived as part of a small community and it focused on minimizing restraints.

Benjamin Rush known as the Father of American Psychiatry was one of the pioneers of occupational therapy. He wrote the book *Medical Inquiries and Observations upon the Diseases of the Mind* (1812).

4. **Period of scientific attitude (1796 AD–1878 AD):** Sigmund Freud proposed the topographical and the structural model of mind. Freud developed psychoanalysis to treat patients. Emil Kraepelin introduced the classification for mental disorders. Dorothea Dix visited the asylums and she recommended the government to take measures to improve the conditions in the hospitals. The term psychiatry comes from the Greek word (*psychē*: 'soul or mind') and (*iatros*: 'healer') was coined by Johann Christian Reil in 1808.
5. **Period of prevention (1885–1960 AD):** In 1908, Clifford Beers wrote a book *'The Mind that Found Itself,'* which explained the pathetic conditions that existed in psychiatric wards during his stay as an inpatient. In 1980, the Diagnostic and Statistical Manual (DSM) of Mental Disorders, published by the American Psychiatric Association, was revised. The National Institute of Mental Health (NIMH) declared the 1990s the Decade of the Brain 'to enhance public awareness of the benefits to be derived from brain research.'

HISTORY OF PSYCHIATRY IN INDIA

Origin of psychiatry as a specialty can be traced in Ancient India. Charaka Samhita was the oldest texts which included aspects of psychiatry.

According to Ayurveda, psychiatry was labeled as bhut vidya which means demonology. Three types of personality was defined namely Satvik (characterized by high intellectual and moral level), Rajasik (high emotionality, passionate nature and impulsiveness) and Tamasik (mental subnormality). Bhagavat Geeta is considered to be probably the first recorded evidence of psychotherapy and counseling.

History of psychiatry in India can be categorized into 4 periods such as:

1. **Precolonial period:** King Ashoka established hospitals for patients with mental illness. According to Ashoka Samhita, these hospitals were built with separate enclosures.
2. **Colonial period (1745–1857):** One of the earliest mental hospitals in India was set up in Mumbai in 1745. First mental hospital at Kolkata was built during the time of Lord Cornwallis in 1787. The credit for the establishment of this hospital goes to Surgeon George M. Kenderline.

First mental hospital was started in Chennai at Kilpauk, in 1794 for 20 patients by Surgeon Valentine Conolly.

Until the early part of the nineteenth century, mental asylums were located only at three major cities and they mostly catered to the British and the Indian sepoys employed by the British. The mentally ill from the general population were taken care of by the local communities and by traditional qualified doctors in Ayurveda and Unani medicine.

3. **Mid-colonial period (1858–1947):** During this period, India witnessed a steady growth in the development of mental asylums. The first Lunacy Act was enacted in the year 1858. Moral treatment for the mentally ill was adopted and implemented during this period.

   Colonel Owen AR Berkeley-Hill, the then superintendent of the European Hospital (Central Institute of Psychiatry, Ranchi) took efforts to raise the standard of treatment and also persuaded the government to change the term 'asylum' to 'hospital' in 1920.

   Health Survey and Development Committee (Bhore Committee) in 1946 surveyed mental hospitals and suggested that more focus has to be taken for the training of personnel and students in psychiatry and promotion of occupational and diversional therapies. One of the proposals put forward by Bhore Committee was the establishment of Department of Mental Health in the proposed All India Medical Institute.

4. **Postindependence period (1947–2000):** Mudaliar committee in 1962 recommended the establishment of independent psychiatric or mental health clinics and institutions for mentally ill. Mudaliar committee also recommended that Ranchi mental hospital has to be converted into full-fledged training institute in addition to All India Institute of Mental Health, Bengaluru.

   By the 1960s, Central Institute of Psychiatry (CIP, Ranchi) and Madras Mental Hospital offered a range of specialized services, including child and adolescent clinics, geriatric, epileptic and neuropsychiatric services. The concept of a day hospital was an important innovation. One of the earliest rural mental health clinics was started at Mandar near Ranchi in 1967.

   On the recommendation of the Bhore committee, All India Institute Mental Health was set up in 1954, which became the National Institute of Mental Health and Neurosciences (NIMHANS) in 1974 at Bengaluru. National Mental Health Program was adopted by the Central Council of Health and Family Welfare, in 1982. The first draft of Mental Health Act that subsequently became the Mental Health Act of India (1987) was written at Ranchi in 1949.

HISTORY OF PSYCHIATRIC NURSING: INTERNATIONAL LEVEL

Florence Nightingale initiated measures to meet the needs of psychiatric patients with proper hygiene, better food, light and ventilation and the use of drugs to restrain aggressive patients in 1840. These efforts contributed to reduction in mortality rate and improvement in the behavior of patients. During the 19th century, as a result of the reform movements, Psychiatric-Mental Health Nursing evolved as a specialty to provide treatment for the mentally ill. The first organized efforts to develop psychiatric nursing started at McLean Asylum in Massachusetts in 1882. Lind Richards was the first trained psychiatric nurse in US. She planned the curriculum for the McLean Training School for Nurses.

Harriet Bailey wrote the first psychiatric nursing textbook, *'Nursing Mental Diseases.'* Jane Taylor was the proponent for the inclusion of Psychiatric Nursing. Psychiatric nursing was included in the general nursing programs at Johns Hopkins Hospital in 1913. Hildegard Peplau published *'Interpersonal Relation in Nursing'* in 1952.

The first doctorate program in psychiatric nursing was started in 1960 in Boston. Maxwell Jones wrote a book on Therapeutic Community in which he emphasized the role of nurse in taking care of mentally ill clients. The American Nurses Association (ANA) developed standard of care in Psychiatric Nursing in 1973, so as to improve the quality of care. Scope and standards of Psychiatric-Mental Health Nursing was published by ANA in 2000.

DEVELOPMENT OF PSYCHIATRIC NURSING IN INDIA

History reveals that during the period of Emperor Ashoka, two male and two female nurses were recruited for the care of mentally ill. The role of the nurses was to meet the basic needs of the patient as well as administration of herbal medication.

During the initial period of establishment of asylums, nurses primarily provided custodial care, in addition to attending the basic physical needs of the patients. During 1919, Berkeley-Hill, the medical superintendent of European Mental Hospital in Ranchi appointed 12 staff nurse and 1 matron from UK and they were given 1 year training. During this time, nurses were involved in the provision of therapeutic environment.

In 1954, orientation course for 4–6 weeks duration for the nurses working in psychiatric units were organized at Nur Manzil Mental Health Center, Lucknow. In 1956, one year post certificate course in psychiatric nursing started in NIMHANS with an annual intake of 20 seats. Duration of Diploma in Psychiatric Nursing was reduced to 11 months in 1975.

In 1965, Indian Nursing Council included psychiatric nursing in GNM and BSc Nursing curriculum. Psychiatric nursing was made as a separate examination by Indian Nursing Council in 2004. In 1975, MSc in Psychiatric Nursing was offered in Raj Kumari Amrit Kaur College of Nursing, New Delhi with an annual intake of 4.

In 1991–1992, the Indian Society of Psychiatric Nurses was registered.

CHALLENGES IN PSYCHIATRIC NURSING

Numerous issues and trends influence the psychiatric-mental health nursing practice. Mental health nurses often encounter a wide variety of challenges which occurs due to demographic, social, economic and technological changes.

- **Demographic changes:** According to WHO, between 2015 and 2050, the proportion of the world's older adults is estimated to almost double from about 12 to 22%. Elderly often face neglect and are subjected to abuse. Older adults most often develop mental disorders. Thus the mental health nurse has to be competent to meet the needs of the elderly. Psychogeriatrics is the branch of psychiatry which deals with behavioral and emotional problems of elderly. Geropsychiatry deals with the treatment of mental illness in elderly.

  Joint family has been replaced by nuclear family. In a nuclear family, family members lack opportunity to disclose their problems and the children also are not getting sufficient attention and care, so they are vulnerable to have mental health problems.
- **Social changes:** Human beings are becoming more conscious of their rights. Increased prevalence of juvenile delinquency and drug abuse are often attributed to peer pressure.
- **Economic changes:** As a result of urbanization and industrialization, people are often under stress to achieve the standard of living. Psychiatric mental health nurse often has to extend their services to the family and community.
- **Technological changes:** Mass media, computers and internet have profound influence on the people. Psychiatric mental health nurse can take a major role in educating the public the issues related to substance abuse, child abuse, adolescent health, family life and care of elderly. Mental health nurses must have knowledge and skill with the new technological advancements, so that she can deliver quality patient care.

TRENDS IN PSYCHIATRIC NURSING

- **Educational preparation of the nurse:** The educational programme for nurses in India which equip to practice as nurses in the field of psychiatry include the following as shown in Table 2.1.

Table 2.1: Educational programs for nurses in India

Course	*Duration*
General Nursing and Midwifery	3 years
BSc (Basic) Nursing	4 years
BSc (Post Basic) Nursing	2 years
MSc Nursing	2 years
M Phil	1 year (Full time) 2 years (Part time)
PhD	3–5 years
Diploma in Psychiatric Nursing	1 year

General Nursing and Midwifery course has 70 hours theory and 8 weeks of clinical experience in mental health nursing. BSC Nursing has 120 hours of theory and 9 weeks of clinical experience. This educational preparation helps the nurse to take up the role of first level care providers in psychiatric mental health nursing setting. MSc Nursing course prepares the student to practice as nurse clinicians. M Phil and PhD equip the students to undertake research in the field of mental health nursing.

- **Standards of psychiatric-mental health nursing practice:** In order to provide quality nursing care and to fulfill the profession's obligations, American Nurses Association has developed the standards of psychiatric nursing.
- **Development of code of ethics:** Code of ethics helps the psychiatric mental health nurse to take up independent role.
- **Involvement of legal issues:** It is important that mental health nurses are to be aware of the rights of mentally ill and legal responsibilities of the nurse.
- **Changes in the role of psychiatric-mental health nurse:** Psychiatric mental health nurse can assume a wide variety of roles which include:
  - *Nurse clinician:* She identifies the emotional and behavioral problems of the client and provides comprehensive care in settings like Neuropsychiatric wards, general hospital, obstetric units, cardiac, burns, surgical unit and geriatric unit.
  - *Nurse therapist:* Role of the nurse therapist is to provide psychotherapy to the client on therapeutic, preventive and promotive approach.
  - *Nurse educator:* Nurse educator has to prepare the students at different level, so as to equip them to provide quality nursing care.
- **Cost-effective nursing care:** Nursing care of good quality with minimum cost has to be rendered.

- **Care to the vulnerable or high risk groups:** Psychiatric mental health nurse has to render care to the vulnerable group which include the children, pregnant women, victims of violence and the elderly.
- **Research:** Nurses have to carry out research activities for implementing quality care.

NATIONAL MENTAL HEALTH PROGRAMME (NMHP)

Mentally ill persons constitute a vulnerable section of society and are often subjected to discrimination in our society. National Mental Health Programme was launched by Government of India in 1982, keeping in view the heavy burden of mental illness in the community and inadequate mental health care services in the country.

India was the first developing country to formulate National Mental Health Programme. The services provided at Sakalwara, Bengaluru and Raipur Rani helped in initial development of NMHP.

Objectives

- To ensure the availability and accessibility of minimum mental health care for all particularly to the most vulnerable and underprivileged sections of the population.
- To encourage the application of mental health knowledge in general health care and in social development.
- To promote community participation in the mental health service development and to stimulate efforts towards self-help in the community.

Aims

- Prevention and treatment of mental and neurological disorders and their associated disabilities.
- Use of mental health technology to improve general health services.
- Application of mental health principles in total national development to improve quality of life.

Strategies

- Integration of mental health with primary health care through the NMHP.
- Provision of tertiary care institutions for treatment of mental disorders.
- Eradicating stigmatization of mentally ill patients and protecting their rights.

Components of NMHP

- Extension of District Mental Health Programme to 100 districts
- Upgradation of Psychiatry wings of Government Medical Colleges/ General Hospitals
- Modernization of State Mental hospitals
- Information, Education and Communication (IEC)
- Monitoring and Evaluation
- Manpower Development Schemes
- Training and Research.

DISTRICT MENTAL HEALTH PROGRAMME (DMHP)

A model for DMHP was initiated by NIMHANS, which is known as Bellary model in 1985. District Mental Health Programme (DMHP) is a part of National Mental Health Programme which provides mental health services in each district. The main objective of DMHP is to integrate mental health with general health services through decentralization of treatment from tertiary level of care to primary health care services. The components of DMHP are early detection and treatment, training, IEC and monitoring.

DMHP was started in Thiruvananthapuram in 1999. DMHP, Thiruvananthapuram has its nodal center functioning at Mental Health Centre, Peroorkada. It focuses on rendering mental health services to the rural areas and creates awareness among the public so as to reduce the misconceptions and to seek services for the early diagnosis and treatment of mental illness.

DMHP Team Members

- Psychiatrist
- Clinical Psychologist
- Psychiatric Social Worker
- Psychiatric Nurse
- Program Manager
- Record Keeper

CONCLUSION

Psychiatry as a branch of medicine deals with thoughts and emotions and thus provides an important platform for promoting the mental health of individual and the society as a whole. The combination of primary health care in mental health care, has led to a shift from the concept of care rendered in hospitals to the one that is rendered at community.

BIBLIOGRAPHY

1. Ahuja N. A Short Textbook of Psychiatry (Seventh edition). New Delhi: Jaypee Brothers Medical Publishers (P) Ltd, 2011.
2. District Mental Health Programme Available from https://dmhptvpm.org/about.html (Accessed on 13 May, 2017).
3. Frisch N, Frisch L. Psychiatric Mental Health Nursing (Fourth Edition). Delmar Cengage Learning, New York, 2011.
4. Halter, Margaret J Varcarolis, Elizabeth M (Eds). Varcarolis' Foundations of Psychiatric Mental Health Nursing: A Clinical Approach. St Louis, Mo: Elsevier, 2014.
5. National Mental Health Programme Available from https://nhp.gov.in/national-mental-health-programme (Accessed on 13 May, 2017).
6. Sadock BJ, Sadock VA, Ruiz P. Kaplan and Sadock's Synopsis of Psychiatry: Behavioral Sciences/Clinical Psychiatry (Ninth edition). Philadelphia: Wolters Kluwer, 2009.
7. Sreevani R. A Guide to Mental Health and Psychiatric Nursing (Third Edition). New Delhi: Jaypee Brothers Medical Publishers (P) Ltd, 2016.
8. Stuart GW, Laraia MT. Principles and Practice of Psychiatric Nursing. St Louis: Mosby, 2001.
9. Townsend CM. Psychiatric Mental Health Nursing: Concepts of Care in Evidence-based Practice (7th Edition). Philadelphia: FA Davis Company, 2012.
10. Vyas JN, Ghimire RS. Textbook of Postgraduate Psychiatry (Third edition). New Delhi: Jaypee Brothers Medical Publishers (P) Ltd, 2016.

CHAPTER 3 Therapeutic Nurse-Patient Relationship

COMMUNICATION

Humans have an innate need to communicate and to relate to others, there by adding worth to personal life. Communication is the foundation stone for initiating and maintaining relationships. Communication is an interactive process between two or more persons who send and receive messages. Communication is very essential component of psychiatric nursing.

Definition

Communication refers to process of imparting, conveying or exchanging of ideas, knowledge, and message among individuals.

Communication is the exchange of information, thoughts and feelings among people using speech or other means (National Institute of Health).

Elements of Communication

Berlo (1960) has explained the components or elements of communication based on SMCR model (Fig. 3.1).

Sender (S)

Person who sends the message is referred to as sender. Sender is also known as encoder or source. The communication skills, language and culture of the sender should be similar to that of receiver.

Message (M)

Idea or information that is sent or received. Idea should be clear and concise.

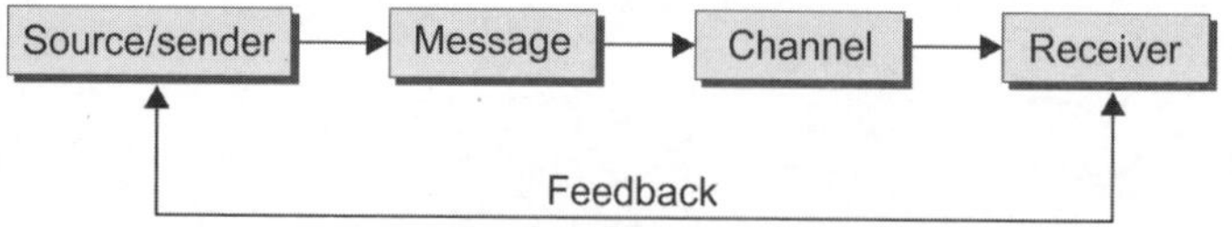

Fig. 3.1: SMCR model depicting the elements of communication

Channel (C)

Media through which the message is sent. Channels of communication used are touch, seeing, hearing, tasting and smelling.

Receiver (R)

Person receiving the message is known as receiver. Receiver is also known as decoder.

Feedback

Response given by the receiver.

Types of Communication

Verbal Communication

Communication which occurs through the use of words, spoken or written. When information or ideas is communicated through words, it is called verbal communication. Verbal communication is of two types: written and oral communication. Face-to-face conversations, group discussions, and E-mail are examples of verbal communication.

Nonverbal Communication

Information or ideas are communicated without the use of spoken or written words is known as nonverbal communication. The types of nonverbal communication include vocal cues, gestures, physical appearance, posture, touch and spacing.

Interpersonal Communication

Refers to the communication between two persons.

Transpersonal Communication

In this type of communication, an individual speaks to God. Prayer, meditation are examples of transpersonal communication.

Intrapersonal Communication

Form of communication in which an individual communicates with oneself. This includes self-talk and inner thoughts.

Factors Influencing Communication

Communication is affected by many factors like attitude, ability of the individual to interact, knowledge, sociocultural background, environmental factors and physical and emotional health (Fig. 3.2).

- **Attitude:** Attitude of a person is determined by various life experiences. If a person is caring and open minded, he will be able to communicate better.

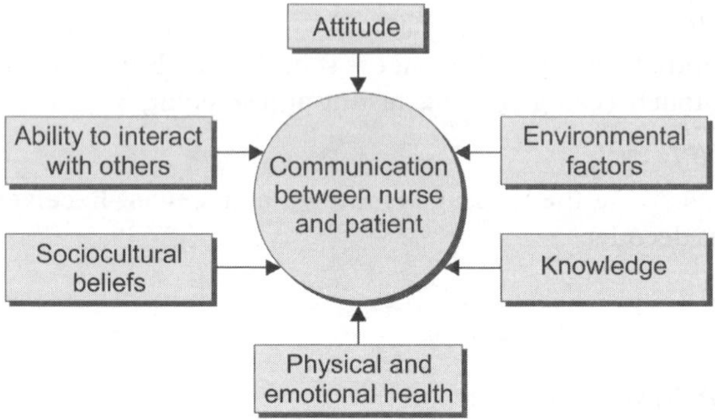

Fig. 3.2: Factors affecting communication

- **Ability of the individual to interact:** Ability to interact is also a learnt behavior from one's own experiences. A person who is able to interact easily with others is able to communicate effectively.
- **Knowledge:** Knowledge of the sender as well as that of the receiver is essential for effective communication. If the receiver is ignorant, he may not understand the idea communicated by the sender.
- **Sociocultural background:** Difference in the customs and beliefs of different societies greatly influence communication.
- **Environmental factors:** Environmental factors like place, time, and noise level often affect the communication.
- **Physical and emotional health:** Communication may not be proper if the persons involved are having severe pain, fatigue or anxiety and fear.

Barriers of Communication

Barriers of communication are shown in Table 3.1.

Table 3.1: Barriers of communication

Physical barriers	• Lack of privacy • Noise • Information overload
Physiological barriers	• Vision impairment • Hearing deficits • Cognitive impairment
Psychological barriers	• Introvert personality • Poor communication skills • Socioeconomic status • Anxiety, fear, sad mood • Poor concentration
Language barriers	• Reduced clarity of message • Use of jargon

Communication Skills

For effective communication, the nurse should possess the following skills:
- Speak clearly
- Avoid using jargon or scientific terminology
- Speak slowly
- Active listening
- Asking open ended questions
- Using silence and pauses
- Observing for the gestures or words.

THERAPEUTIC COMMUNICATION

Refers to an interpersonal interaction between the nurse and the client for promoting the physical and emotional health of a client. Therapeutic communication occurs when the nurse communicates to the patient in such a way that brings out a therapeutic outcome.

Purposes of Therapeutic Communication

- Help the client express their ideas and feelings.
- Fosters the client's comfort.
- Promotes a feeling of safety, and increases their trust in the nurse.

Techniques of Therapeutic Communication

Nurses use therapeutic communication techniques to offer support and provide information to clients. Variety of communication techniques can be used to accomplish nursing goals while interacting with a client (Table 3.2).

Table 3.2: Techniques of therapeutic communication

Sl. no.	*Types of therapeutic communication*	*Description*	*Purpose*	*Example*
1.	Broad opening	The conversation is focused directly on the client	Helps to initiate a conversation. Provides an opportunity to express his feelings	How do you feel?
2.	Using general leads	Use of verbal communication or through facial expression and nodding	Helps to direct the conversation. Motivates the client to communicate further	O'I see Ok, go on Uh, hm

Contd...

Contd...

Sl. no.	*Types of therapeutic communication*	*Description*	*Purpose*	*Example*
3.	Active listening	Nurse listens actively to the client.		Characteristics of active listening are: • S-Sit facing the client • L-Lean forward • O-Open posture • R-Relaxed
4.	Restating	Repeats the main ideas revealed by the client	Conveys that the nurse is listening	'I don't like to go to college because I don't like the teacher' Nurse restates 'You don't like to go to the school as you don't like the teacher'
5.	Reflecting	Repetition of client's statement as a whole or a part of by the nurse	Validates the information	Client—'Everyone dislikes me' Nurse—'Dislikes you?'
6.	Sharing observations	Observations made by the nurse is shared with the client	Helps to validate her observations	'You are restless'
7.	Focusing	Expanding the conversation on the topic of importance	Provides more clarity and focuses on reality	'We will talk more about the issues with your husband'
8.	Using silence	Nurse reduces the pace of conversation	Helps the client to collect his thoughts and speak further	Sitting quietly along with client
9.	Giving information	Information regarding the disease is rendered by the nurse	Helps to develop trust in the nurse-client relationship	'Schizophrenia occurs due to the increased amount of certain chemical substances in the brain'
10.	Clarifying	Nurse clarify the feelings or ideas expressed by the patient	Helps to prevent misunderstanding Demonstrate the interest of the nurse over clients feelings	'I am not clear about the main issue here'

Contd...

Contd...

Sl. no.	*Types of therapeutic communication*	*Description*	*Purpose*	*Example*
11.	Exploring	Collect more details about topics which the client has put forward for discussion	Helps to get a complete awareness of the topic	'Tell me more about that', 'Would you describe it more fully?'
12.	Presenting reality	When the client misinterprets reality, the nurse can present the real fact	Useful in geriatric clients, psychiatric clients having high anxiety and those who are confused due to alcohol or drugs such as LSD	'I am not hearing any sound' 'Your father is not here; he is your cousin.'
13.	Voicing doubt	Express uncertainty as to the reality of the client's perceptions	Provides an opportunity for the client to be aware that others do not necessarily perceive facts in the same manner	'Is that you have said really happened?' 'It's very difficult to believe.'
14.	Suggesting	Presenting a variety of alternatives and allow the client to choose one of them		Two alternatives are existing for your problem. You can decide which one suits you best
15	Summarizing	Highlights the important information that has been discussed	Helps to clarify the information given	'So far we have discussed the ill effects of alcoholism'
16	Humor		Promotes feelings of closeness and friendliness	
17	Asking relevant question	To obtain needed information	Help to explore over the area of concern	'What is the major problem troubling you'

Nontherapeutic Communication Technique

Nontherapeutic communication techniques include those communication techniques that interfere with professional relationships.
Nontherapeutic communication techniques include:
- Asking personal questions
- Giving personal opinions
- Changing the subject
- False reassurance
- Sympathy
- Asking for explanation
- Approval or disapproval
- Arguing.

PROCESS RECORDING

Process recording is a tool which records the interaction between the nurse and the client. It is a written record or verbatim recording of all that occurred during the nurse-client interaction.

Purposes of Process Recording

- Used as an educative tool—to educate the students regarding the communication.
- Used as a diagnostic tool—aids in identifying the symptoms of the client.
- Used as therapeutic tool—it aids in improving the communication and social skills of the client.

Objectives of Process Recording

Process recording helps in achieving the objectives for the student nurse as well as for the client.

Objectives for the Student

- Identify the symptoms of the client.
- Establish rapport with the client.
- Helps in analyzing the communication techniques and interpersonal relationship.

Objectives for the Client

- Helps in improving communication and interpersonal skills.
- Assists in developing insight.
- Contributes to therapeutic outcome.

Sample for Process Recording

Identification Data

Name of the Client —Mr Z
Age —21 years
Ward No —Ward 10
Marital status —Unmarried
Occupation —Student
Date of Admission

Chief Complaints: According to client

'I tried to commit suicide'

According to Informant

- Loss of sleep × 2 weeks
- Loss of appetite × 2 weeks
- Suicidal ideations × 3 days
- Suicidal attempt × 1 day

Present Psychiatric History

Mr Z was apparently normal 2 weeks back. Two weeks before he had loss of sleep, he used to sleep hours in the night, remaining time he used to sit lonely in his room. He also had poor appetite; he used to take small quantity of food two times in a day. For the past 3 days, he is expressing suicidal ideations. One day before admission, he tried to commit suicide by hanging. So the relatives brought him to mental health center.

Introductory Remarks

- Appearance of the client including his behavior: He was poorly groomed, looking dull
- Setting of the interaction: Ward 10
- Date
- Time and Duration: 10-10.30 am, 30 minutes.

Objectives for the Student

- Establish rapport with the client.
- Identify the symptoms of the client.
- Helps in analyzing the communication techniques and interpersonal relationship.

Objectives for the Client

- Helps in improving communication and interpersonal skills.
- Assists in developing insight.

Table 3.3: Recording and analysis of the verbatim

What the nurse said and did	*What the client said and did*	*Therapeutic technique used*	*Analysis of the client's response*
N- Hai, Good morning, I am nursing student and I would like to talk with you. Would you like to speak with me, Rajesh	P-Good morning, Sister (he wishes back) P-No problem	Giving recognition Offering self	Normal posture Willing to initiate conversation
N- Had your breakfast?	P-Yes, sister		
N-What you had in the morning?	P- I had two dosa and chutney. Now my appetite has improved	Broad opening	Recent memory intact
N-How do you feel now? (Leaning forward, making eye contact)	P- I am happy (looks without any emotion)	Broad opening	Subjective mood happy Affect is blunt and incongruent
N-Why are you admitted here?	P- My family consists of father, mother and brother. They do not like me. So I wanted to end my life.	Asking questions	Insight present
N- You said you really wanted to kill yourself?	P- Yes, I felt really sad I was no longer able to handle the situation. I felt I am not an useful person and there is nobody to help me	Restating	Ideas of worthlessness and helplessness
N- However, it is a good thing that you recognized your suicidal thoughts and sought treatment. Still you are having thoughts of harming self?	P-Not now, I have a lot of worries and I would like to be in a group	Clarifying	Accepts the suggestion
N-Whether you would like to participate in a therapy group where you could ventilate your feelings	P-Yes, I really want to be member of the group	Suggesting	He is motivated to attend the therapy session
N-Participation in a therapy group will help you a lot to handle difficult situation	P-Thanks for listening to me and for the information given	Information giving	He acknowledges the information shared

Contd...

Contd...

What the nurse said and did	*What the client said and did*	*Therapeutic technique used*	*Analysis of the client's response*
N-So far we had a brief interaction regarding your concerns and I have suggested for participation in therapy groups. I wish that you will have better strength in dealing with your problems. See you at the same time on the next day	P-Ok, Bye	Summarizing	He agrees to attend the therapy session

Summary

Mr Z was poorly groomed and looking dull. Rapport was established. His mood was happy. He had ideas of worthlessness and hopelessness. His immediate memory was intact. Therapeutic communication techniques used were giving recognition, offering self, broad opening, asking question, restating, clarifying, suggesting, information giving and summarizing. He was ready to accept the suggestions given.

THERAPEUTIC NURSE-CLIENT RELATIONSHIP

Therapeutic nurse-client relationship is the foundation of all psychiatric nursing treatment measures. It is important that the nurse should enter into relationship that is confidential, safe and consistent.

Definition

Therapeutic nurse client relationship is an interpersonal process between the nurse and the client to help client (Rawlin).

It is a time bound alliance between the nurse and the client which is consciously entered and characterized by empathy, respect, acceptance and genuineness.

Types of Relationship

There are two types of relationship—social relationship and therapeutic relationship.

Differences between therapeutic relationship and social relationship are depicted in Table 3.4.

Table 3.4: Differences between therapeutic relationship and social relationship

	Therapeutic relationship	*Social relationship*
Definition	It is a time bound alliance between the nurse and the client which is consciously entered and characterized by empathy, respect, acceptance and genuineness.	Relationship that is primarily initiated with the purpose of friendship, socialization, enjoyment or accomplishing a task.
Responsibility	One person takes the responsibility of helping the other person.	Persons are not in position of having responsibility.
Purpose	There is a specific purpose.	The specific purpose is not necessary.
Goal direction	It is goal directed.	It is not goal directed.
Nature of the relationship	Relationship is entered through necessity.	Relationship is entered by choice.
Duration	Definite and anticipated ending.	Relationship may continue indefinitely.

Components of Therapeutic Relationship

- **Empathy:** Empathy is the ability of the nurse to perceive the feelings of the client and to convey that understanding to the client. It is the ability to put oneself in another person's feeling. Empathy is different from sympathy. Sympathy is the sharing of other person's emotions. For example your friend tells you that her father is diagnosed to have cancer, and then your empathetic response would be "Tell me about your thoughts and feelings" and you stay with the friend and help her to cope with the situation (Fig. 3.3).

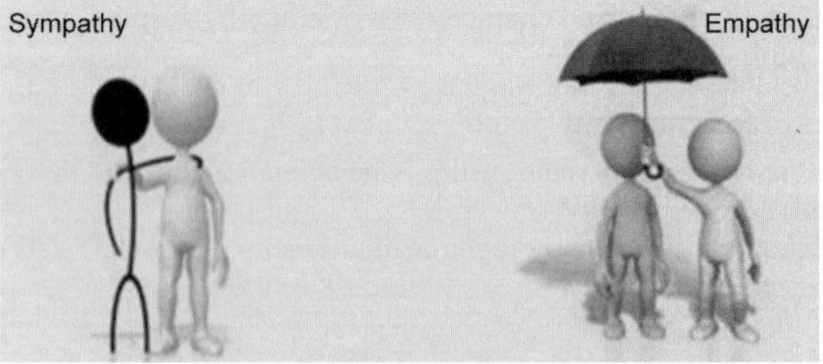

Fig. 3.3: Comparison between empathy and sympathy

- **Warmth:** It is the ability to help the client feel cared for and comfortable. It shows acceptance of the client as a unique individual.
- **Genuineness:** Refers to the true feelings of the nurse while providing care to client. It is ability of the nurse to be aware of one's own thoughts, feeling and values and apply this in the immediate interaction of the client. Here the nurse honestly explains facts to the client.
- **Rapport:** It is the willingness to be involved with other person. When rapport develops the client feel comfortable with the nurse and finds it easier for self-disclosure.

Goals of Therapeutic Nurse-Client Relationship

- **Helps in the identification of client problem:** Nurse-client relationship provides an opportunity to identify his problem in a realistic manner. Example: A woman who shows violence finds out that her violence is due to the abuse from her alcoholic husband.
- **Helps the client to identify his role in his behavior:** Nurse can help the client to be aware of his behavior and once he suggests a remedy, he can be made clear about his ability to take appropriate decision.
- **Helps the client to cope with the problem:** Nurse collects data regarding the client's problem and also his past coping methods and thus helps him to cope up with his problem.
- **Helps the client to find out new solution for his problem:** During her interaction with the client, nurse finds out that he has used possible ways to overcome a problem, but failed. So the nurse helps the client to understand that many alternate solutions exist and he has to select the best one.
- **Assists the client to adopt new patterns of behavior:** Nurse identifies that the client has certain maladaptive behavior, so the nurse helps to adopt a new pattern of behavior. Example: A client is not communicating, so the nurse encourages him to talk to another person in the ward. Once he talks, nurse gives positive reinforcement for his new behavior.
- **Assists the client to communicate:** Mentally ill clients often have problems in communication. Some may not communicate, while others may display increased speech.
- **Helps the client to socialize:** Mentally ill clients often have poor social interaction. In such situation, nurse can assist the client for improving socialization. Nurse has to determine the appropriate time for initiation of socialization. She can first engage client in one-to-one interaction and later on progress to one-to-many interactions.

Factors Affecting Therapeutic Nurse-Client Relationship

- **Self-awareness:** Refers to the process of understanding one's own beliefs, thoughts, abilities and limitations. Self-awareness includes self-concept, beliefs, values and life experiences. Self-concept includes all that one knows about himself. Nurse's beliefs and values will influence the nurse-client interaction and also nursing care. Life experiences of the nurse will most often affect the nursing care rendered.
- **Attitude towards the client:** Nurse should have a positive attitude towards caring mentally ill. Mentally ill client develops trust only if nurse accept him as a unique individual.
- **Rapport:** Rapport is defined as relation of harmony and accord between the client and health care provider (Dorland's Medical Dictionary). Three qualities required for establishing rapport are warmth, genuineness and empathy.

PHASES AND STAGES OF NURSE-CLIENT RELATIONSHIP (PEPLAU'S INTERPERSONAL THEORY)

The phases of nurse-client relationship can be categorised into 4 phases (Fig. 3.4):

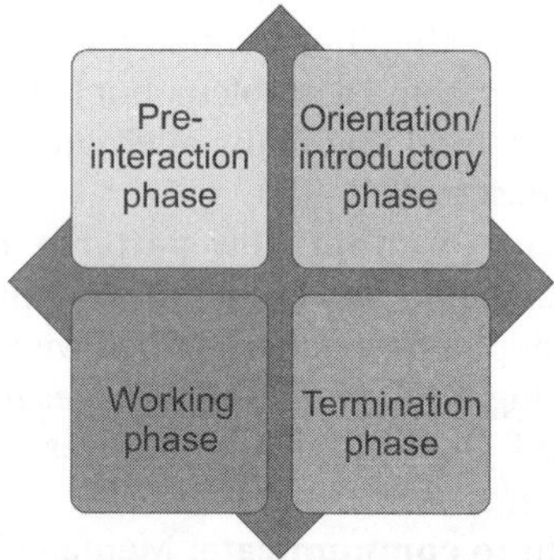

Fig. 3.4: Phases of nurse-client relationship

Preinteraction Phase

Refers to the phase which begins when the nurse is assigned to initiate a therapeutic relationship. During this phase, nurse collect details regarding the client from the case record or other health care providers in the concerned ward. The nurse may experience fear and anxiety regarding the initial interaction with the client.

Task Involved during the Preinteraction Phase

- Explore one's own feelings and fear.
- Gathers data about the client.
- Plan for the first meeting with the client.

Barriers during the Preinteraction Phase

- **Difficulty in exploring one's own feelings and fear:** During the preinteraction phase, nurse tries to identify her own feelings towards meeting the client. At the same time, nurses find it difficult to explore her own feelings.
- **Anxiety:** Before the initial meeting with the client, nurses often experience anxiety and fear. Factors contributing to nurse's anxiety include fear of communication or fear of assault from the client.

Ways to Overcome Barriers during the Preinteraction Phase

During the preinteraction phase, nurse can talk about her anxiety to friends as well as to the clinical supervisor. Nurses can formulate goals for the initial interaction and can prepare a plan for the meeting.

Orientation Phase/Introductory Phase

Refers to the phase during which the nurse meet the client for the first time. This is the starting phase for the entire therapeutic interaction.

Tasks of the Orientation Phase

- Establish trust and acceptance.
- Establish communication.
- Identify the problems.
- Sets goals/objectives for the interaction.
- Establish a nurse-client contract or pact.

During this phase once the trust is established, client talks with the nurse regarding his problems. Once the problems are identified, nurse and the client formulate goals for the interaction. The nurse makes a pact or agreement with the client which contribute to a therapeutic outcome. It is important that confidentiality has to be ensured.

Elements of Nurse-Client Contract

Elements of nurse-client contract are given in Table 3.5.

Table 3.5: Elements of nurse-client contract

• Name of the nurse and the client
• Explanation of the objectives
• Responsibility of client
• Date, time and place of the meeting
• Meeting conditions for termination

Barriers during the Orientation Phase

- **Perception of the client and the nurse:** The client may perceive the nurse as an important person in his life. Transference is the unconscious transfer of qualities associated with another individual to the nurse by the client. Example—If the client perceives the nurse as his granddaughter, then he starts behaving as her grandfather, it is a type of transference.

  Two types of transference:
  1. **Hostile:** The client become critical and irritable to the nurse.
  2. **Dependent:** Regards the nurse as a God like figure.

     Similarly the nurse may consider the client as an important person in her life. Counter transference is the unconscious transfer of qualities originally associated with another individual to the client by the nurse. Example—If the nurse perceives the client as her mother, then nurse provides care as if she is her mother, it is a type of counter transference.

     Types of counter transference are intense love or caring, intense hostility or intense anxiety.
- **Difficulty in establishing the nurse-client contract:** Client often feels that nurse is incompetent or time is inadequate to achieve the set objectives. Anxiety of the nurse as well as he client may also act as a barrier during the orientation phase.

Ways to Overcome Barriers during the Orientation Phase

Discussing with the supervising teacher will help to resolve the barriers during this phase.

Working Phase/Exploitation Phase

Working phase is the phase during which nurse and the client work towards attainment of goals formulated during the orientation phase. During this phase the nurse will be implementing the nursing actions. It is the action phase of the relationship.

Task of the Working Phase

- Gather further data.
- Help the client to identify his problems.
- Assist the client to initiate communication.
- Motivates the client to socialize.
- Promotes socialization skills.
- Help to identify problem-solving skills.
- Encourage to adopt new patterns of behavior.
- Evaluate the problems, goals and redefine.
- Prepares the client for the termination of relationship.

Barriers during the Working Phase

Testing of the Nurse by the Client

Clients often test the knowledge and skills of the nurse. A client with aggressive behavior may attempt to provoke the nurse to determine whether or not she will take some disciplinary action.

Progress of the Client

The condition of the client may act as barrier during the working phase. When the client's symptoms improve with the rendered nursing care, nurse feels more confident. But if the client's condition deteriorates during the working phase, nurse feels incompetent.

Stressful Life Events of the Nurse

When the client explains his life events, nurse who has experienced the same may be using her own problem-solving strategies.

Resistance Behavior by the Client

Client sometimes display some resistance behavior like not revealing the relevant data, showing anger or irritability, acting out or terminating the relationship.

Ways to Overcome Barriers during the Working Phase

Nurses can overcome the above mentioned barriers by having discussion with the supervisors and with other staff members. The nurse has to improve listening skills so as to reduce resistance behavior of the client.

Termination/Resolution Phase

This phase refers to the termination of the nurse-client relationship. This is the most difficult phase of nurse-client relationship. During the interaction phase itself, nurse has to make client convince the estimated time of relationship.

Criteria for Determining the Termination of Nurse-Client Relationship

- Client experiences relief from presenting problems.
- Client's social function has improved.
- His ego function is strengthened.
- Completion of student nurses clinical experience.

Task in the Termination Phase

- Have a therapeutic end to nurse-client relationship.
- Establish the reality of separation.
- Review the progress of therapy and attainment of goals.
- Formulate plans.
- Mutually explore feelings of rejection, loss and sadness.

Barriers during the Termination Phase

- **Fault finding:** Clients are often not ready to terminate the relationship. They try to find fault in whatever things nurse do and often blames her for fault.
- **Resistance:** Client often is reluctant to disclose his problems to the nurse. Résistance behavior includes suppression of inner conflicts or exaggeration of symptoms.

Ways to Overcome Barriers during the Termination Phase

Clients often feel deserted on termination of relationship. Nurse has to allow the client to openly express his thoughts and feelings related to termination. Nurse should explore her feelings and thoughts regarding the separation from the client. When planning for discharge, nurse also has to prepare herself for termination of relationship. The supervisor can help the nurse to initiate measures to prepare both self and client.

THERAPEUTIC IMPASSES

Therapeutic impasses are factors that hinder in the progress of nurse and client relationship. Therapeutic impasses provoke anxiety, frustrations or intense anger in the nurse and client.

Types of Therapeutic Impasses

- Resistance
- Transference
- Counter transference
- Boundary violations.

Occurs when the nurse violates the limits of therapeutic relationship and establishes a social relationship with the client. Boundary violations can occur in the following areas:

- **Space:** The nurse should not allow the client to enter her personal space.
- **Place:** Nurse should not plan a meeting with the client out of hospital.
- **Time:** Nurse should not plan a meeting with the client at odd times.
- **Appearance:** Appearance of a nurse should be simple.
- **Gift:** Nurse should avoid giving and taking gifts from the client.

Management of Therapeutic Impasses

- Nurse should develop self-awareness.
- Avoid self-disclosure.
- Encourage the client to openly express his feeling and thoughts.
- Discuss with supervisors.

CONCLUSION

Nurse-client relationship is vital for all nursing practice. Each interaction in nurse-client relationship is unique as it involves two individuals—nurse and the client who differ in their beliefs, values and attitudes. Knowledge, attitude and communication skills of the nurse are important factors required for establishing an effective nurse-client relationship.

BIBLIOGRAPHY

1. Berman TA, Snyder S, Kozier JB, Erb G. Kozier and Erb's Fundamentals of Nursing (8th Edition). London: Pearson, 2007.
2. Communication in Nursing Practice-NCBI-NIH. Available from https://www.ncbi.nlm.nih.gov Accessed on April 2017.
3. Dorland Dorland. Dorland's Illustrated Medical Dictionary (32nd Edition). Elsevier, 2011.
4. Kapoor B. Textbook of Psychiatric Nursing. Delhi: Kumar Publishing House, 2014.
5. Potter, Thomas, Sharma. Fundamentals of Nursing (South Asian Edition). India: Elsevier, 2013.
6. Rawlins PR, Williams RS, Beck KC. Mental Health-Psychiatric Nursing: A Holistic Life-Cycle Approach. St Louis: Mosby, 1998.
7. Shives RL. Basic Concepts of Psychiatric-Mental Health Nursing. Philadelphia: Lippincott Williams & Wilkins, 2008.
8. Sreevani R. A Guide to Mental Health and Psychiatric Nursing (Third Edition). New Delhi: Jaypee Brothers Medical Publishers (P) Ltd, 2016.
9. Stuart GW, Laraia MT. Principles and Practice of Psychiatric Nursing. St. Louis: Mosby, 2001.
10. Theodore DD. Textbook of Mental Health Nursing. India: Elsevier, 2015.
11. Townsend CM. Psychiatric Mental Health Nursing: Concepts of Care in Evidence-Based Practice (7th Edition). Philadelphia: FA Davis Company, 2012.

CHAPTER 4

Mental Health Assessment

INTRODUCTION

Assessment is the first component of nursing process. This includes systematic collection and analysis of data collected from patients and their relatives.

TECHNIQUES OF MENTAL HEALTH ASSESSMENT

The basic techniques of mental health assessment include:

- Psychiatric history.
- Mental Status Examination (MSE).
- Mini Mental Status Examination (MMSE).
- Medical investigations.
- Psychological tests.

Psychiatric History

This allows the psychiatric nurses to determine the course of illness.

Objectives of collecting history

- Provide an opportunity to identify the predisposing factors and causes of mental illness.
- Helps in identifying the symptoms of the client.
- Aids in formulating nursing diagnosis.
- Assists in planning and implementing nursing interventions.
- Helps the client and relatives to express feelings.

Psychiatric history can be organized under the following headings:

Demographic Data

This should include the name, age, education, occupation, marital status, address, date of admission and source of referral.

Informant Details

Include details regarding the source of information, relationship of the informant to the patient and period of stay with the patient. Reliability and adequacy of the information also has to be obtained.

Presenting Chief Complaints with Duration

- **Patient version:** Record it in patient's own words with adequate description
- **Informant version:** Record the complaints along with its duration in a chronological order. Include the major disturbances in the different areas of functioning.

History of Present Illness

This provides a comprehensive and chronologic picture of the events leading to current symptoms. Give a detailed account of the symptoms from the onset of the symptoms, till the admission or consultation.

Specific attention must be paid to the following:

- **Onset:** Record the onset of the symptoms, whether it is abrupt (within 48 hrs), acute (within 1 week), subacute (1–2 weeks), insidious (few weeks–few months), chronic (more than 6 months).
- **Course of the illness:** The course of an illness can be episodic (discrete periods with symptoms with intervening periods of normal behavior), continuous or fluctuating (periodic exacerbations of a continuous illness).
- **Precipitating factors:** Enquire about any precipitating events. These could be physical (e.g. a febrile illness), psychological in nature (e.g. death/loss) or pharmacological (non-compliance to drugs).
- **Associated disturbances:** Enquiry should also be made regarding the impairment in other areas of functioning-disturbances in sleep, appetite, weight, sexual life, social life and occupation.

Past History

This includes information regarding past psychiatric illness, medical and surgical history.

History of Past Psychiatric Illness

Details regarding total duration of illness, initial onset of symptoms has to be obtained. Record the nature and duration of symptoms and the treatment received during each episode of illness.

History of Past Medical-Surgical Illness

Information has to be collected for any history of medical or surgical events like fever/trauma/headache/vomiting/confusion/disorientation/memory disturbances/neuropathy/head injury/meningitis/encephalitis/epilepsy/delirium/typhoid/TB/syphilis .

Family History

The description should include information of family members as whether they are living or dead, age, education, occupation, marital status and relationship with the patient. Describe the socio-economic status of the family. Enquire about any psychiatric illness, delinquency, personality problems, suicide, substance abuse, epilepsy, mental retardation or any hereditary medical illnesses.

Family history may be presented in the form of family tree (genogram) and it should have three generation (Figs. 4.1 and 4.2).

Personal History

Birth and Early Development History

Antenatal Period: Obtain details regarding the physical and psychiatric problems of mother during pregnancy, any exposure to radiation or use of drugs.

Intranatal Period: Whether the baby was born full-term/premature/ postmature, mode of delivery, any complications during delivery, whether the baby cried immediately after delivery. Birth weight of the baby, birth defects—if any.

Postnatal Period: Include details regarding any postnatal complications like cyanosis/convulsions/jaundice. Whether mother had psychiatric problems during the postpartum period.

Childhood History

Ascertain whether child has attained developmental milestones at appropriate age or not.

Behavior and Emotional Problems: Enquire about sleep disturbances, thumb-sucking, nail-biting, temper tantrums, bed-wetting, stammering,

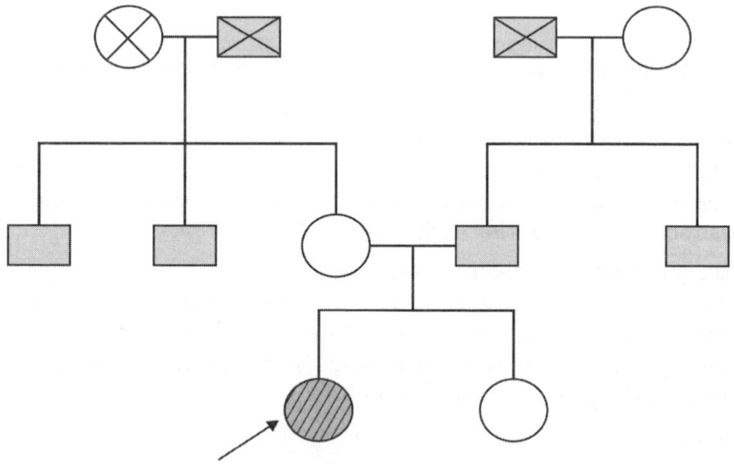

Fig. 4.1: Example for a family tree

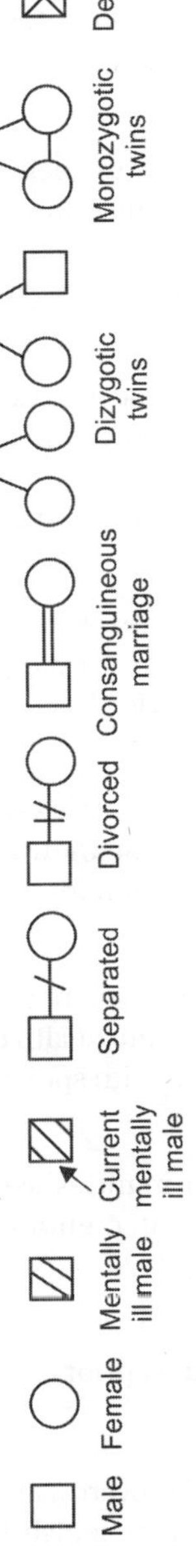

Fig. 4.2: Symbols in a family tree

tics, mannerisms/attention deficits/impulsivity/disobedience/fears/ worrying/lack of self-confidence/attention seeking behaviors.

Emotional Problems during Adolescence: Record if there is history of running away from home/delinquency/smoking/drug taking.

Educational History

Obtain information regarding age at the beginning of formal education, academic performance, educational status, any failures, reason for failure, academic and extracurricular achievements, peer relations, disciplinary problems, discontinuation/change of school.

Occupational History

Record the details including age at starting the work, jobs held in chronological order, frequent changes in jobs, reason for changes, present job and income, job satisfaction, promotions/awards, relationship with colleagues, superiors and subordinates.

Menstrual History

Enquire about age of menarche; reaction to menarche, regularity of periods; associated physical and psychological symptoms to current cycle and LMP (Last Menstrual Period).

Sexual History

Record the age at appearance of secondary sexual characteristics anxiety related to puberty changes, source of knowledge regarding sex, history of sexual abuse and premarital/extramarital sexual relations.

Marital History

Obtain details with regard to the type of marriage, age at the time of marriage, age/education/occupation/health of the partner at marriage, interpersonal and sexual relations with spouse.

Obstetrical History

Number of children, any abnormalities associated with pregnancy, delivery and puerperium, age at menopause and any associated problems has to be recorded.

Premorbid Personality

In this description of the personality prior to the beginning of the mental illness has to be included. Premorbid personality is assessed in the following aspects:

- **Interpersonal relationships:** Introvert/extrovert
- **Attitude to self:** Positive/negative, selfish/thought to others
- **Attitude to others:** Positive/negative, selfish/thought to others

- **Attitude to work and responsibility:** Decision making power, acceptance of responsibility, flexibility.
- **Use of leisure time:** Hobbies/interest/intellectual activity/energetic/sedentary
  - *Predominant mood*: Optimistic/pessimistic/stable/fluctuating/cheerful/despondent.
- Reaction to stressful events
- Religious belief and moral attitudes
- Habits
  - Eating pattern
  - Elimination
  - Sleep
  - Use of drug, tobacco, alcohol, other psychoactive substances.

Psychoactive Substance Use History

In case of patients who are using psychoactive substance, it is important to collect information like age at first use, cause of first use, history of dependence, history of withdrawal symptoms, reason for re-starting, maintaining factors, money spent for daily use.

Mental Status Examination (MSE)

Mental status examination is an assessment of general motor behavior, thought, emotional functioning along with evaluation of judgment and insight.

Major components of MSE include:

- General appearance and behavior
- Psychomotor activity
- Speech
- Thought
- Mood
- Perception
- Cognitive functions
- Judgment
- Insight.

General Appearance and Behavior

As the part of general appearance, observe the appearance, body built, hygiene, grooming, posture and gait.

Appearances include the way the patient is dressed in terms of time, place and occasion. Body built is noted as ectomorphic/mesomorphic or endomorphic. See whether the patient maintained personal hygiene or not. Posture is the position assumed by the patient at the time of examination. It can be closed posture (patient is sitting with the legs crossed, hands put on the chest and looking down) or an open posture (patient sits confidently and maintains eye to eye contact) or may have normal erect posture. Gait should be recorded as staggering, small steps or walks normally.

Behavior is assessed through observation of facial expression, eye to eye contact and gesture. Mode of entry for the mental status examination, rapport, attitude towards the examiner and presence of hallucinatory behaviors should also be noted.

Psychomotor Activity

Observe the psychomotor activity - whether it is increased, decreased or normal. Assess for any other psychomotor abnormalities like tics/ stereotyped movements, mannerisms, gestures, restlessness, agitation, aggressiveness, rigidity, echopraxia and negativism.

Speech

- A neutral topic can be given to the client so as to elicit the characteristics of speech, e.g. a festival/rain/sea.
- Note the initiation of speech, reaction time (the amount of time taken to elicit an answer).
- Is the amount of speech is little or minimal or excessive? Is the speech is high toned or low toned?
- Is the speech relevant?
- Is it coherent?
- Observe for any speech abnormalities (rhyming/punning/echolalia/ perseveration/neologism/clang association).

Thought

Thought has to be assessed in the areas of form and stream, content and possession.

- **Form and Stream:** Note whether form of thought is normal and assess for the presence of thought disorder. Abnormalities in the form of thought includes neologism/flight of ideas/clang association/ glossolalia/word salad specify with a sample of speech. See whether the stream is normal/abnormal. Abnormalities in the stream of thought includes loosening of association/circumstantiality/ tangentiality/thought block/retardation of thinking/preservation.
- **Content**: Specific questions can be used to elicit different types of delusions.
  - Delusions of - grandiose/persecutory/nihilistic/infidelity/love/ somatic/ hypochondriacal/ poverty/ guilt/ bizarre.
  - Preoccupations, depressive ideation (worthlessness, helplessness, and hopelessness), suicidal ideas, phobias, obsession and compulsion must be recorded.

- **Possession**: Thought alienation—ask questions to elicit thought insertion/thought broadcasting/thought withdrawal.

Mood

Assessment of the mood has to be done both subjectively and objectively.

Subjective evaluation is done by asking the client 'How do you feel?' or 'How is your mood?'

Description should be given regarding the range of affective responses,- congruity (in relation to thought processes) and appropriateness (in relation to situations).

Perception

Record the presence of illusions and hallucinations. Enquire about hallucination in the following modalities—vision, hearing, smell, touch, taste. With respect to auditory hallucinations include details whether the hallucinations are first person, second person or third person and content of hallucinatory voices.

Cognitive Functions

Consciousness

Assess the level of consciousness of patient . This may range from alert, confused, clouding of consciousness, stupor and coma.

Orientation

Orientation is assessed in terms of time, place and person.

Orientation to time can be assessed by asking questions—what is the time now?/Is it morning, afternoon, evening or night? Or what is the day today?

Orientation to place and person is elicited by asking place and by asking him to identify his relatives or family members.

Memory

Assessment of memory is done in the areas of immediate, recent and remote memory.

- Immediate memory: Tested by digit span test or by recalling the names of 3 unrelated objects like apple, fan and car after 5 minutes.
- Recent memory: Tested by asking—the date of admission or what he has taken for breakfast or dinner? or by asking the patient to recall events in the last 24 hours.
- Remote memory: Ask about information on life events like—date of birth and age, date of marriage or time since marriage or death of any family member, year of completing education.
  (verify all the answers with the relative).

Attention

Tests used to elicit for attention in clinical situation is Digit Span test - which include Digit forward and Digit backward tests.

- Forward: Patient is given the following instructions:
  'I will be saying some digits, listen to me carefully and repeat them in the same order, when I finish it, e.g. : If I say 3, 7 you say 3, 7.'

  Similarly, read the digits at the rate of one digit per second to the patient and note the immediate response of the patient- whether it is said correctly or not.

  The following digits may be used:

5-7-3	4-1-2
5-3-8-7	6-1-8-4
2-9-7-3-4	6-1-5-8-3
7-2-5-9-4-8	4-7-1-5-3-8

The same digits should not be presented more than once

If the patient cannot repeat a particular number of digits on one trial, a 2nd trial can be done with the same number of digits and credit is given if the response is correct.

- Backward: The patient is instructed as follows:
  'I will be saying some digits, listen to me carefully and repeat them after me in a reversed order, for example: if I say 2-5. You have to say 5-2.'
  The procedure is the same as that of digit forward, by using different numbers, but instruct to say in the reverse order.
  Digit backward score is the highest number of digits correctly recalled backward after a maximum of 2 trials.

Concentration: (Normally sustained/distractible).

Serial Subtractions: The examiner instructs the patient to subtract the following series—serial ones, serial threes and serial sevens and notes the time taken in seconds.

Task:	**Correct response and the time limit**
20 to 0	reversed in 15 secs.
40-3 series (5 digits)	40, 37, 34, 31, 28 in 60 secs.
100-7 series (5 digits)	100, 93, 86, 79, 72 in 120 secs. (Note the answers and time taken)

Days or Months Backward: Patient can also be instructed to tell the days of a week/months in a year in the reverse order.

Intelligence

This includes the areas of general information and arithmetic.

- General Information: Ask questions that are relevant to the patient's literacy.

For an illiterate person, ask—5 colors, fruits, flowers, three seasons/festivals and their months. For educated persons, ask the name of Prime Minister/Chief Minister, 5 rivers or 5 states, Capitals of countries.

- Arithmetic ability:
  The following questions may be asked :
  Simple arithmetic calculations like:
  $7 + 5 = ?$, $9 - 3 = ?$, $6 \times 3 = ?$, $6/2 = ?$
  Or
  - How much is 3 rupees and 5 rupees?
  - Suppose you have bought 5 pens of 5 rupees cost and paid a 100 rupees note. How much is the price for 5 pens ? How many rupees balance you have to get ?

Abstract Thinking

It is tested by Proverb test and Similarity and Dissimilarity test.

- Proverb test is done by:
  - Asking the patient to say a proverb.
  - Then ask him about the meaning of that proverb.
  - If patient is unable to say a proverb, examiner can ask the meaning of proverbs like –
    - 'All that glitters are not gold'
    - 'Slow and steady wins the race'
    - 'Barking dog seldom bite'
    - 'All that white are not milk'
- Similarity and dissimilarity test is done by asking the similarities and dissimilarities of -
  - Apple and Orange (Similarity - Both are fruits, Dissimilarities are in color and in taste)
  - Eye and Ear (Similarity - Both are sense organs, Dissimilarity is that eyes are for seeing and ears are for hearing).

The response of the patient is to be noted verbatim and judged to be correct/incorrect.

Judgment

It is assessed in the following areas:

- Personal Judgment
  It is assessed by asking about the patient's future plans.
- Social Judgment
  It is assessed by observing behavior in social situations or his behavior in ward.
- Test Judgment

For assessing it, the following 2 problems are presented to the patient-

- Fire problem: Ask 'If the nearby house catches fire, what is the first thing you will do?'
  (Correct answer—Try to put it off with water and call for help/ fire force).
- Letter problem: Ask 'If you see a stamped and sealed envelope with address on your way in the roadside, what will you do'?
  (Correct answer—Post it in a letter box or give it to the postman).

Insight

This tests the patient's level of awareness of his illness.
Grading of Insight is as follows:
Grade I: Complete denial of illness.
Grade II: Slight awareness of being sick, need help but denying it at the same time.
Grade III: Awareness of being sick but blaming it on an external factors or organic factors.
Grade IV: Awareness that illness is due to something unknown in patient.
Grade V: Intellectual insight.
Grade VI: True emotional insight.

PHYSICAL EXAMINATION

A complete physical examination with system wise assessment and special emphasis on neurological assessment is mandatory.

Summary

The purpose of a summary is to provide concise description of all the important aspects of the mental status examination so as to reach a conclusion. The summary should be presented in the same format/ order as described in the previous pages.

Formulation

It should always include a discussion of the diagnosis - the etiological factors and clinical features which seems to be important, a plan of management and an estimate of the prognosis, regardless the uncertainty or complexity of the case, a provisional diagnosis.

Diagnosis should always be specified using the International Classification of Diseases (ICD).

Mini Mental Status Examination

It is a standardized screening tool for assessing cognitive impairment like dementia. It is shortened version of mental status examination. This test evaluates orientation, registration, concentration, language, short-term memory and visual-spatial concept. This test can be done in 10 minutes and maximum score is 30 point.

Scoring

24–30 Normal, 18–23 Mild to moderate cognitive impairment and 0– 17 Severe cognitive impairment. (See Appendix for Mini MSE format)

Medical Investigations

Routine Investigations

- Hemogram, urinalysis
- Renal function test
- Liver function test
- Serum electrolytes
- Blood glucose
- Thyroid function test
- Serum creatine phosphokinase (CPK)
- Electrocardiogram (ECG)
- Chest X-ray.

Electrophysiological Tests

Electroencephalogram (EEG) helps in assessing electrical activity of brain and to diagnose seizure disorder and degenerative changes of brain.

Polysomnography

It is used in seizure and sleep disorders.

Radiological Investigations

- Computed tomography (CT scan)
- Magnetic resonance imaging scan (MRI scan)
- Positron emission tomography (PET)

Neuroendocrine Tests

- Dexamethasone suppression test
- Thyroid releasing hormone stimulation test
- Serum melatonin levels.

Psychological Tests

Psychological tests are used in the assessment of personality pattern, intelligence, psychotic features and other symptoms of psychiatric disorders. It is being done by an experienced clinical psychologist and accurate interpretations are contributing much to diagnosis and treatment.

Interview in Psychiatric History Collection

Interview is a planned conversation with a purpose of getting or giving information or for identifying problems or for giving support.

Psychiatric history collection is a nondirective interview which helps in rapport building.

Interview questions can be closed questions, open ended questions or neutral one. But in psychiatric assessments open ended questions will be useful in exploring thoughts and feelings, to change topic and to assess attitudes. This will help in getting descriptive answers.

Example: What is the reason for present admission?

Closed questions can be used wherever necessary, e.g. How old are you? Where are you working?

Neutral questions are also relevant in history collection, e.g. How do you feel now?

Interview Setting and Technique

Existing health problems, present complaints and other available information can be reviewed before beginning the interview. Consider the factors that can influence interview—Time, Place, Seating arrangement and Language.

- **Time:** Interview must done when the patient is comfortable and cooperative. Get consent and cooperation of family members/informant. Time should be scheduled to prevent interruption from other professionals, and thus privacy can be ensured. Time should be planned based on the convenience of patient and family.
- **Place:** A medium sized well-lighted and ventilated room with no noise and interruptions should be selected. Avoid the presence of other people in the room to ensure confidentiality. This will facilitate free interaction.
- **Seating:** Seating arrangement must be done with adequate spacing—two to four feet apart and a table in between. When client is in bed, seating can be at 45 degree angle to the bed. Distance between nurse and patient or family member should not be too smaller or greater.
- **Language:** Nurse must communicate in simple clear language, according to the level of understanding of patient and relative.

Always begin the interview with greeting and self-introduction from the part of nurse. Start with casual talk that conveys your concern. Once patient/relative shows an attitude of acceptance, enter the topic of concern, based on objective of interview. Get detailed information, by being active listener and with empathizing approach. Do not hurry up or look at watch. Terminate the interview by a conclusion and by thanking the patient and family member. Relevant points can be noted then and there.

CONCLUSION

Assessment has important role in mental health nursing. Psychiatric patients usually deny their illness due to lack of insight. Nurse's observations, history collection, mental status examination, evaluation of investigation reports and prompt reporting can improve the quality of care.

BIBLIOGRAPHY

1. Ahuja N. A Short Textbook of Psychiatry (Seventh edition). New Delhi: Jaypee Brothers Medical Publishers (P) Ltd, 2011.
2. Genogram Symbols—Genopro Available from https://genopro.com/genogram/symbols/Accessed on June 25 2017.
3. Kapoor B. Textbook of Psychiatric Nursing. Delhi: Kumar Publishing House, 2014.
4. Kozier B, Erb G, Snyder S. Fundamentals of Nursing: Concepts, Process and Practice (Seventh edition). Delhi: Pearson Education, 2004.
5. Sadock BJ, Sadock VA, Ruiz P. Kaplan and Sadock's Synopsis of Psychiatry: Behavioral Sciences/Clinical Psychiatry (Ninth edition). Philadelphia: Wolters Kluwer, 2009.
6. Sreevani R. A Guide to Mental Health and Psychiatric Nursing (Third Edition). New Delhi: Jaypee Brothers Medical Publishers (P) Ltd, 2016.
7. Townsend CM. Psychiatric Mental Health Nursing: Concepts of Care in Evidence-Based Practice (7th Edition). Philadelphia: FA Davis Company, 2012.

CHAPTER 5

Psychopathology of Mental Disorders

PSYCHOPATHOLOGY OF MENTAL DISORDERS

Introduction

Psychopathology simply means the study of pathology of mind. It deals with disturbance of human behavior that occurs as a part of disorders of thought, emotion and perception and other cognitive functions.

Definitions

Psychopathology is the study of psychological and behavioral dysfunction that occur in mental illness. Scientific study of mental disorders that include etiology, classifications, manifestations and treatment of psychiatric disorders.

Review of Anatomy and Physiology of Brain

Review of structure and functions of brain will help the student nurse in better understanding of psychopathology.

Human brain is the central organ of central nervous system and it controls all our activities by integrating and coordinating the information received from different sense organs. Brain and spinal cord together is called central nervous system.

Brain is divided into three major areas—Cerebrum, Brain stem and Cerebellum.

Parts of Brain, their Functions and Correlation to Mental Disorders (Figs 5.1 and 5.2)

Parts of brain, their functions and correlation to mental disorders are given in Table 5.1.

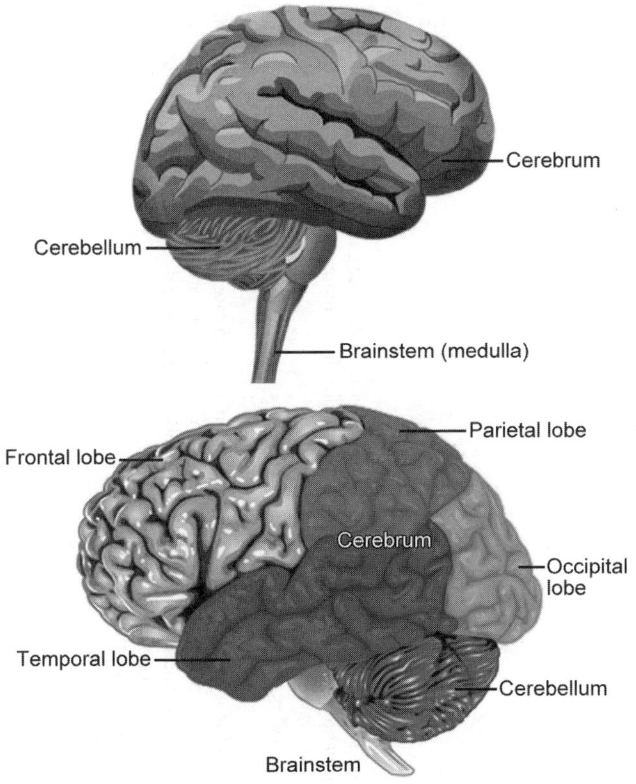

Fig. 5.1: Parts of brain

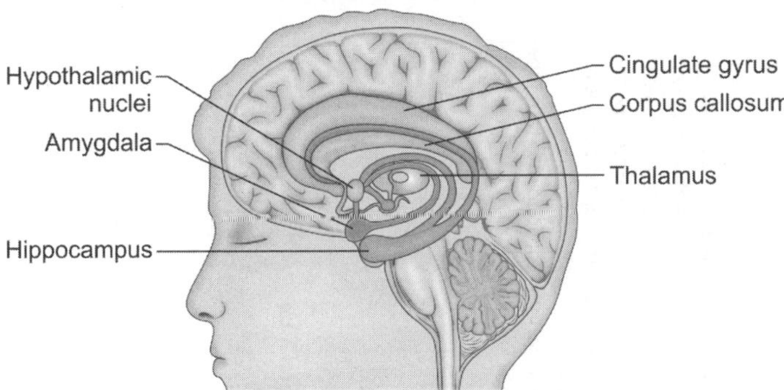

Fig. 5.2: Limbic system

Table 5.1: Parts of brain, their functions and correlation to mental disorders

Parts of brain	*Functions*	*Dysfunction*
Cerebrum It is the largest part that forms about 80% of the weight of brain. Cerebrum is divided into right and left hemispheres that are covered by cerebral cortex. Here the inner white matter is covered by an outer layer of grey matter. Each hemisphere is divided into four lobes —Frontal, Parietal, Temporal and Occipital lobes		
1. Frontal lobe	Frontal lobe is concerned with thinking, reasoning, planning and executive functions, general motor functions and motor aspects of spoken and written speech	Changes in frontal lobe can lead to fear, irritability, aggression and sometimes depression or apathy
2. Parietal lobe	It is the area of sensory functions of taste, temperature, pain perception, and memory association, sensory speech. Another important function is proprioception which is the position sense of body. Left parietal lobe is associated with language interpretation	Dysfunction can cause inability of sensations – pain, touch, temperature, inability to learn from past, inability to understand spoken or written words

Contd...

Contd...

Parts of brain	*Functions*	*Dysfunction*
3. Temporal lobe	It is the site of memory, learning, abstract thinking and judgment. It plays a role in smell perception and expression of emotions, due to connectivity with limbic system. Left temporal lobe is usually dominant and involved in language processing, complex memory and emotional stability	Temporal lobe has important roles with abnormal perceptions like illusions and auditory hallucinations. Increase or decrease in the activity of left lobe can lead to labile emotions, aggressive or violent thoughts that lead to homicidal or suicidal activity
4. Occipital lobe	Main function of this lobe is visual perception and interpretation (responsible for understanding written words and images)	Involved in visual hallucinations. Impairment in visual memory Inability to understand written words
Limbic system (Fig. 5.2) It is formed by portions of frontal, parietal, and temporal lobes that form a continuous ring like band of cortex around the top of brain stem. Other parts of limbic system are Amygdala, Hippocampus, Cingulate gyrus, Nucleus accumbens, Thalamus and Hypothalamus	It is the reward center of brain that motivates us to do or learn something that gives satisfaction. It is also called 'Emotional brain' and is responsible for emotional responses like anger, anxiety, fear, pleasure, sadness and sexual feelings. Limbic system is concerned with motivation, emotion and memory	
Amygdala	It is involved in control of emotions by coordinating the actions of autonomic nervous system and endocrine system. It is essential for nurturing behavior and fear conditioning	Dysfunction of amygdala leads to inappropriate fear, anxiety, hyperactivity or attention deficit and post-traumatic stress disorder

Contd...

Contd...

Parts of brain	*Functions*	*Dysfunction*
Hippocampus	It is the information processing center between the parts of brain that receive sensory experiences and areas that translate these experiences to action. It has role in regulation of immune system	Any damage or malformation of this area is usually lazy and may resist learning due to the difficulty in recalling the learned information
Cingulate gyrus	It has role in regulation of stress response, the emotional content of physical pain. It is the link between motivation and behavior	
Nucleus accumbens	It is the exact reward center of brain. Decreased dopamine receptors in this area leads to marked decrease in the ability to experience pleasure It is the site where psychoactive substances like cocaine, nicotine, amphetamine, alcohol, marijuana have their action	
Thalamus	It is the relay station and processes almost all sensory and motor information that comes from spinal cord, cerebellum and brainstem	Dysfunctions in thalamus lead to difficulty in the interpretation of pain. It is also involved in schizophrenia, obsessive compulsive disorder and mood disorders

Contd...

Contd...

Parts of brain	*Functions*	*Dysfunction*
Hypothalamus	It is an integration center that converts thoughts and feelings into hormones which leads to physical changes through autonomic nervous system. It also regulates autonomic nervous system by involving in water balance, maintenance of blood pressure, sleep, appetite, temperature	Dysfunction of hypothalamus will lead to excessive thirst and hunger. It is involved in anorexia nervosa and bulimia nervosa
Brainstem Brainstem consists of midbrain, pons and medulla. Vital centers – centers of respiration, heart rate, balance and blood pressure are located here. Other tiny structures in brainstem are – raphe nuclei, locus coeruleus and substantia nigra	Raphe nuclei are the primary source for serotonin in the brain and spinal cord. Locus coeruleus is located in the pons and is the primary source of norepinephrine. Stimulation of this area causes instant fear response Substantia nigra is the main source of dopamine for the brain	Degeneration of dopamine cells in the substantia causes motor dysfunction in Parkinson's disease
Cerebellum Cerebellum coordinates the timing of skeletal muscle contractions in movement. It helps in maintenance of posture and equilibrium in association with inner ear. It is concerned with procedural memory		Procedural memory (performance of tasks like brushing, buttoning) will be impaired can occur in case of cerebellar dysfunction. Difficulty in acquiring motor skills, impairment in regulation of movement, inability to walk straight and problems with balance

Neurotransmission

It is the process that allows the electrochemical transmission of nerve signals from one neuron to another at synapse. As impulse travels from neuron through the axon, storage vesicles will release the stored neurotransmitters which act as the chemical messenger.

Electrical impulses release neurotransmitters from the presynaptic neuron into the synaptic cleft. Based on the type of neurotransmitter, the receptor cells are stimulated or inhibited. Once this transmission is over, the neurotransmitter is reuptaken to the presynaptic neuron and stored for future use or it will be inactivated by enzymes.

Neurotransmitters

Neurotransmitters are endogenous chemicals that transmit signals from a neuron to a target cell across a synapse.

Being the chemical messengers in impulse transmission, they have important role in functions of brain and thus human emotions and behavior.

Table 5.2: Classification of Neurotransmitters

Neurotransmitters are broadly categorized as:
• Cholinergics – Acetylcholine • Monoamines Catecholamines – Dopamine – Epinephrine – Norepinephrine Histamine Classical Tryptamines – Serotonin – Melatonin • Amino acids – GABA (Gamma-Aminobutyric Acid) – Glutamate • Neuropeptides – Substance P – Neurotensin – L-tryptophan – Galanin – Cholecystokinin

Functions and Dysfunctions of Neurotransmitters

Functions and dysfunctions of neurotransmitters are shown in Table 5.3.

Table 5.3: Functions and dysfunctions of neurotransmitters

Neurotransmitter	*Functions*	*Correlation with mental disorders*	
		Excess	*Deficit*
Acetylcholine	Learning and memory Emotional regulation Socialization Exploration Motor function Sleep and arousal	Anxiety, somatic complaints and depression	Disorder of memory, Disorder of motor behavior, Antisocial behavior, Alzheimer's disease, Parkinson's disease
Dopamine	Motor activity long-term memory thinking, decision making, integration of thoughts and emotions	Schizophrenia and mania, Disorganized thinking, Loosening of association, Tics and stereotypic behavior	Parkinson's disease and depression Movement disorders Poor impulse control
Epinephrine and Norepinephrine	Regulation of cognition- alertness, attention, orientation Learning and memory Regulates energy, appetite and mood Fight or flight response	Mania, Anxiety states Hyperalertness leading to anxiety and panic attack Loss of appetite Increased energy Sensation seeking behavior	Depression Low energy and dullness
Histamine	Involved with allergic reactions and sexual behavior	Little is known about its role in mental disorders	
Serotonin (5-HT)	Regulation of mood and emotional behavior Anti-impulsive action (Inhibition and calmness in activities) Regulation of sleep cycle Precursor to melatonin that is concerned with circadian rhythm	Schizophrenia Sedation Increased sleep Decreased anxiety, sex drive Severe increase cause hallucinations	Irritability, Insomnia, Anxiety, Depression, poor impulse control and Suicidal tendency

Contd...

Contd...

Neurotransmitter	*Functions*	*Correlation with mental disorders*	
		Excess	*Deficit*
GABA (Gamma-Aminobutyric Acid)	Slows down the activities of body (inhibitory neurotransmitter) Regulates anxiety Influence muscular coordination Role in cognition, memory and reduction of aggression	Sedation, Impairment in recent memory	Anxiety disorders, movement disorders and epilepsy. Irritability Lack of coordination of movement
Glutamate	Excitatory neurotransmitter Learning and memory development and strengthening of synapse	Epilepsy Alzheimer's disease	Increase of symptoms in schizophrenia

ETIOLOGY OF ABNORMAL BEHAVIOR IN PSYCHIATRIC DISORDERS

Behavior is considered as normal or abnormal based on the social norms and customs.

A single factor cannot be pointed out as the cause of mental illness. Multiple factors are involved in this and in general they can be divided as predisposing, precipitating and perpetuating factors.

- **Predisposing factors:** These are the factors that predispose, or make the individual more susceptible to mental illness. Genetic factors along with adverse psychosocial factors will make one more susceptible to mental illness. Any illness or injury to central nervous system also may predispose to abnormal behavior.
- **Precipitating factors:** These are the life events that have occurred prior to the onset of a disorder.
  Example: Death of near one, Loss of job, Failure in exam.
- **Perpetuating factors:** These are the factors that aggravate or prolong the duration of an existing illness in the individual.
  Example: Physiological changes in pregnancy and postpartum period can aggravate an existing mental illness. Sometimes a primary cause may be there, without which the disorder would not have occurred, e.g. head injury leads to abnormal behavior.

CAUSES OF MENTAL ILLNESS

Biopsychosocial Factors

Specific etiology of mental illness includes biopsychosocial factors. But the etiological theories will be different for each mental disorder.

A. Biological factors: These are the factors related to bodily functions and include:

- **Heredity/Genetic factors:** Inherited genes can predispose the offsprings to mental illness. One third of psychotic people have history of mental disorder in their siblings or in the first degree relatives.

  Example: 14.2% of siblings of schizophrenia patients develop it. But in general population, the prevalence is 0.85% only.
- **Constitutional factors:** It includes body built or physique. People with certain physique are more prone to specific mental illness.

  Example: Endomorphic persons have more chance to develop mania.
- **Physical deprivation:** Malnutrition and sleep deprivation over a long period can cause mental disorder.
- **Biochemical factors:** Dysregulation of neurotransmitters in the brain plays a vital role in the etiology of psychiatric illness. We cannot point out a single neurotransmitter as the specific cause in any of the illness. But some of them have dominating role in specific psychiatric disorder.

  Example: Dopamine has major contribution in development of psychotic features in schizophrenia. Norepinephrine and serotonin has major role in mania and depression.

  But current findings point out that mental disorders are associated with alterations in several neurotransmitters.
- **Neuroanatomical changes (Brain damage):** Any structural damage of brain will affect its functioning and can lead to abnormal behavior that indicate mental illness. Structural changes in brain may occur due to:
- *External causes* (Exogenous *factors*)
  - Infections (HIV infection, Encephalitis, Neurosyphilis)
  - Injury - head trauma
  - Intoxication (drugs, alcohol, lead, etc.)
  - Vitamin deficiency (B complex deficiency, prolonged malnutrition)
- Endogenous Factors
  - Brain tumors
  - Vascular changes (leads to hemorrhage or ischemia)
  - Brain dysfunction due to hypoxia, electrolyte imbalance, alterations in blood glucose level)

- Degenerative changes in brain (dementia).
- Endocrine disorders like hypothyroidism/hyperthyroidism.
- Acute or chronic physical illness that causes disability and thus affects various aspects of life. This can lead to depressive symptoms.

- **Physiological changes:** Changes that occur in specific developmental stages cause psychological changes and sometimes psychological problems. So the chances for mental illness are more in these periods (puberty, pregnancy, postnatal period, menopause, ageing).

B. Psychological factors: Biological factors and psychological problems when occur together, it can precipitate mental illness. Common psychological factors are:

- **Strained/Faulty relationships:** Strained relations at home, work place, schools and colleges, Broken family/marital disharmony among parents, lack of good interpersonal relationship among family members.
- **Grief or Loss:** Loss of loved one, loss of job and prestige, financial loss, etc. are some situations that increases stress.
- **Childhood insecurity** from maternal deprivation, parent's personality problems
- **Faulty parenting**
  - Neglect or over concern from the parents
  - Over strictness or over leniency
  - Lack of love and concern
  - Lack of appreciation
  - Deprivation of psychological and social needs
  - Cruel punishment
  - Unhealthy comparison
  - Lack of play, recreation and socialization.
- **Marriage related problems:** Forced marriage, incompatibility in education, occupation and financial and social status, lack of children, personality problems in a partner, etc.
- **Misconcepts and unhealthy attitude to sex:** This includes premarital and extramarital relationships, sexual perversions promiscuity. These can be due to improper sex education, watching pornography or by being victims of sexual abuse.
- **Stress:** Stressors in daily life include changes or challenges that need special attention to solve. Here the individual feels indecisive and frustrated and will feel difficulty in adjusting. Stressors can precipitate mental illness in the absence of adequate support system. Stressors can cause psychosomatic disorders also.
- **Specific personality pattern:** People with specific personality pattern develop mental illness more easily, e.g. people with schizoid personality are more prone to develop schizophrenia while facing extreme stressors.

C. Sociocultural factors: Environmental factors also add the risk of mental disorders. They are:

- **Social problems:** Unemployment, poverty, insecurity, social discriminations, prejudice, war and violence.
- **Social changes:** Urbanization, migration, industrialization, change in family structure, development of newer technology, change in value system, etc.
- **Social crisis situations:** Natural calamities may lead to psychological problems.

CLASSIFICATION OF MENTAL DISORDERS

Classification of mental disorders or psychiatric taxonomy is an important and basic aspect for all mental health professionals. In the absence of clear etiology, the classification of mental disorders is very difficult.

Presently there are two well-known and widely accepted systems in the classification of mental disorders. They are international classification of diseases (ICD) and diagnostic and statistical manual (DSM). Latest versions of these are ICD 10 and DSM-5:

International Classification of Diseases 10th revision (ICD 10): This is the classification by WHO (World Health Organization) in 1992. It classifies all diseases and related health problems including psychiatric disorders. Chapter 'F' of ICD 10 contains the classification of mental disorders—'mental and behavioral disorders' and it is coded in an alphanumeric system from F00 to F99. There are several versions of ICD10 as:

- Clinical descriptions and diagnostic guidelines (CDDG)
- Diagnostic criteria for research (DCR)
- Multiaxial classification version
- Primary care version.

ICD 10 Mental and Behavioral Disorders

F00-F09	Organic including symptomatic, mental disorders (includes delirium, dementia, organic amnestic syndrome and other organic mental disorders)
F10–F19	Mental and behavioral disorders due to psychoactive substance use (includes intoxication, harmful use, dependence and withdrawal states of substances and psychotic disorders due to substance abuse)
F20-F29	Schizophrenia, schizotypal, and delusional disorders
F31-F39	Mood (Affective) disorders
F40-F48	Neurotic, stress related and somatoform disorders

F50-F59	Behavioral syndromes associated with physiological disturbances and physical factors
F60-F69	Disorders of adult personality and behavior
F70-F79	Mental retardation
F80-F89	Disorders of psychological development
F90-F98	Behavioral and emotional disorders with onset usually occurring in childhood and adolescence
F99	Unspecified mental disorder

Diagnostic and statistical manual of mental disorders (DSM-5): It is the classification by American Psychiatric Association (APA). The latest edition of DSM-5 was released in May 2013.

DSM-5 has three sections:
1. **Section I:** Introduction and instructions to use this new version
2. **Section II:** Diagnostic categories
3. **Section III:** Conditions that need additional research, glossary and important information.

Some important features of DSM-5 are:
- **Nonaxial documentation approach:** There is no more multiaxial assessment system in DSM-5. Previous version (DSM IV) had 5 axes as:
  I. Clinical syndrome/disorders
  II. Personality disorder/mental retardation
  III. Medical conditions
  IV. Psychosocial and environmental stressors
  V. Global assessment of functioning.

The first three axes (I, II, III) combined, and separate notations for the other two axes—psychosocial and environmental factors (IV), and disability (V).
- **New diagnoses are added** (e.g. disruptive mood, dysregulation disorder, hoarding disorder, binge eating disorder, excoriation disorder).
- **Some diagnoses are revised** (e.g. autism spectrum disorder, post-traumatic stress disorder, pedophilic disorder, substance use disorder, specific learning disorder).

Indian Classification

Major classifications in India are done by Neki (1963), Wig and Singer (1967), Vahia (1961) and Varma (1971). It is a modification of ICD 8 classification.

Three main classes are there—psychosis, neurosis and special disorders.

Psychosis

- Functional psychosis (Schizophrenia)
- Affective psychosis (Mania and depression)
- Organic psychosis (Acute and chronic)

Neurosis

- Anxiety neurosis
- Depressive neurosis
- Hysterical neurosis
- Obsessive compulsive disorder
- Phobic neurosis.

Special Disorders

- **Childhood disorders:** Conduct disorders and emotional disorders.
- **Personality disorders:** Sociopath, psychopath
- **Substance abuse:** Alcohol and drug abuse
- **Psychophysiological disorders:** Asthma, psoriasis
- **Mental retardation:** Mild, moderate, severe, profound.

SYMPTOMATOLOGY

Signs and Symptoms of Mental Illness

Signs and symptoms will be different in many psychiatric disorders, and sometimes many of the symptoms are overlapping among them. Most of the psychiatric patients are not reporting their problems, or often deny them. So it is essential for the nurses to have thorough knowledge about the clinical features of mental disorders. Vigilant observations and early detection can contribute much to the care of these patients.

Abnormal behavior in psychiatric disorders may occur in many forms as:

- Disturbance in personality pattern
- Disorders of motor activity
- Disorders of thought
- Disorders of speech
- Disorders of perception
- Disturbance of emotions
- Disorders of consciousness
- Disorders of attention and concentration
- Disorders of orientation
- Disorders of memory
- Disturbance in intelligence
- Disturbance in judgment
- Insight.

Along with these there will be some physical manifestations also.

Disturbances in Personality Pattern

As the part of mental illness, changes may occur in the personality of the individual. For example an introvert may become extrovert and vice versa. People with some personality patterns or traits are more predisposed to some mental disorders.

Example: People with melancholic traits: Features (calm and quiet, kind and sympathetic, good tempered, perfectionists, and preoccupied with work, afraid of failure, feels indecisive and insecure, easily cry alone and suffer in silence) are more predisposed to depression.

Example: People with schizoid personality traits: Features (feel lonely, isolated, shy and asocial but usually good at school. They feel inferior and will not mingle with opposite sex. They are not concerned with their family, and about his personal appearance, but daydreams a lot. Usually disobedient and aggressive during adolescence) are prone to develop schizophrenia.

Example: People with cyclothymic temperament: Features (extreme mood swings, with alternating periods of cheerfulness and sadness) are predisposed to bipolar mood disorder.

Disorders of Motor Activity

Motor activity reflects one's wishes, motivations and instincts and usually is well-coordinated and purposeful.

Disorder of motor activity occurs as disturbance in activity level, or disturbance in qualitative aspects.

Problems with Activity Level

- **Hyperactivity:** Means increased motor activity which is usually seen in hypomania and mania. Here activity is usually goal directed, but because of lack of attention and hyperactivity it could not be finished. Other problems related to hyperactivity are:
  - *Impulsivity:* Means lack of forethought or acting before thinking. Individual is not able to think about the consequences of his/her action.
  - *Restlessness:* Inability to remain still and seems to be active with generalized increase in body movement.
  - *Agitation:* Severe anxiety with motor restlessness. It is seen in many mental disorders.
  - *Excitement:* Emotionally aroused state along with disorganized hyperactivity—(increased speech, with senseless motor activity and hypervigilance).
- **Hypoactivity/under activity/motor retardation:** Activity level is decreased and individual takes too much time to start and complete an activity. It is seen in depression and in some types of schizophrenia.

Quality Disturbance in Motor Activity

- **Tics:** Involuntary repetitive, movement of short duration due to contraction or twitching of small groups of muscles—usually of face or extremities. It is seen as blinking or as strange expressions and sometimes as sniffing, throat clearing or shrugging of shoulders. Tics may occur as single or multiple.
- **Mannerisms:** Habitual gestures or styles of performing normal activities but seems abnormal due to repetition and exaggeration. These movements are usually characteristic of that individual (e.g. scratching the nose or head). Odd mannerisms are characteristic of schizophrenia.
- **Tremor:** Rhythmic oscillatory movements (head or limbs) that occur at rest or with movement.
- **Stereotypy:** It is a spontaneous, purposeless, repeated, regular, uniform movements, but not related to a stimulus.
- **Negativism:** It is motiveless resistance to stimulus either actively or passively. Actively means, individual does the opposite of the command or stimulus. It is seen in catatonia and expressed as mutism or resistance to any passive movement.
- **Automatism:** Automatic performance of activities without conscious knowledge of the patient.
- **Echopraxia:** Repetitious mimicking of actions that are observed. Individual imitates of movements or actions of the examiner or the repetition of simple actions they observe, e.g. mimicking hand movements like clapping.
- **Compulsion:** It is an urge or uncontrollable impulse for repeated performance of an act which are unpleasurable to viewers and individual himself.

Disturbances of Posture and Expression

Posturing is a voluntary assumption of odd posture of body.

- **Catatonia:** It is the disturbance in muscle tone and activity, without any organic basis.
- **Waxy flexibility (Cerea flexibility):** It is the motor disturbance—where person's body is placed and maintained in a particular position, though it is uncomfortable, till it is changed by an external force. Parts of the body seems to be flexible like wax , and this will end in catalepsy.
- **Catalepsy:** Disturbance of posture, in which the individual continuously maintain an immobile position, with rigidity, followed by loss of consciousness.
- **Catatonic stupor:** Severe retardation of motor activity and other responses, leading to immobility and lack of awareness of surroundings.

- **Catatonic posturing:** Voluntary assumption of odd posture that is maintained for long period of time.

Disorders of Thought

Normal thought process is goal directed, and progress in a related manner, so that there will be an association between the matters or content. Thought is expressed in speech. Hence we are taking sample speech for analysis of thought.

Thought disorders are of four types:

1. Disturbances in form and flow of thinking.
2. Disturbance in continuity.
3. Disturbance in content.
4. Disturbance in possession.

Disturbance in the Form and Flow of Thought

Pathological thinking and speech can be very slow or very much increased.

- **Psychomotor retardation:** When the slowness of thought and movement occur together, it is called psychomotor retardation (seen in depression and hypothyroidism).
- **Thought blocking:** Sudden loss of an idea accompanied by the feeling that thought is being taken away from his mind or it is being stolen.
- **Pressure of speech:** Speech and thought occurs at a rapid rate (seen in hypomania, thyrotoxicosis and in some intoxications of caffeine, cocaine.
- **Flight of ideas:** Rapid racing of thoughts in which the rate of speech is extreme rapid, with leaping from topic to topic—but the association in speech is maintained.

Disturbance in Continuity/Progression of Thought

- **Circumstantiality:** Indirect speech with delay in reaching the central point, due to unnecessary/trivial explanations but gradually reaches the original point or desired goal (beat around the bush).
- **Tangentiality:** Here the thought wanders away from the topic and never come back to the main theme.
- **Perseveration:** Repetition of words or sentences beyond the point of relevance as if the person is stuck with that word, e.g. if we ask the patient's name, he/she will answer correctly, but will repeat the same for subsequent questions also.
- **Stereotype speech:** It is the repetition of a word, irrespective of the context.

- **Loosening of association:** It is a pattern of speech in which thought is without any logical relation with one another. It is a primary symptom or a typical thought disorder in schizophrenia.
- **Incoherence:** Thought that is not generally understandable—running together of thoughts or words which are not logically connected and results in disorganized speech. Also called disconnected thinking.
- **Word salad:** Incoherent mixture of words and phrases. That is words that have no logical connection are stringed together.
- **Verbigeration:** Senseless repetition of words that are not understandable.
- **Clang association:** This is a sequence of thought/speech, stimulated by sound of preceding word, and occurs in a rhyming manner, e.g. I met a wet pet set in a net and let it get bet and went to the end.
- **Echolalia:** Repetition of sentence used by the examiner, like a parrot, e.g. if you tell the patient 'Sit there', he/she will repeat it like a parrot.
- **Palilalia:** Repetition of the last word or phrase alone is called palilalia.
- **Neologism:** New word created by the patient, often from combining syllables of other words.

Disorders of Content of Thought

- **Overvalued idea:** Maintenance of unreasonable, sustained false belief, but less firm than delusion.
- **Fantasy:** Vivid imagination with unfulfilled wish as content, but at the same time it is perceived as unreal by the individual.
- **Idea of reference:** False belief, that casual events, people's remarks, etc. are referring to oneself, e.g. while walking on a road, individual believes that others are looking at and talking about him.
- **Obsession:** Pathological persistence/recurrence of an irresistible thought or feeling/idea/impulses, that cannot be eliminated from consciousness due to its intrusive nature. This is associated with anxiety/distress.
- **Phobia:** Persistent, irrational, exaggerated and pathological fear of some specific type of stimulus (thing, situation or activity), resulting in avoidance of the feared stimulus.

Delusions

False fixed belief, not consistent with patient's intelligence and cultural background, that cannot be corrected by reasoning or logical thinking.

Classification of Delusions

- **Based on Origin:**
  - **Primary delusion:** False fixed belief with no definite preceding or precipitating events, e.g. patient has sudden revelation that his relatives have plans to kill him for his property.

- Secondary: False fixed belief that is gradually formed in the light of some early happenings.

- **Depending on Organization:**
  - **Systematized:** Delusions are well organized and confined to a specific area and with several interrelated beliefs that are logically woven.

  Example: If the patient has grandiosity, he may develop delusion of persecution and reference along with this.
  - **Nonsystematized:** These are fragmented and poorly organized and extend to many areas of life.
- **Depending on the Theme of Delusion:**
  - **Delusion of persecution:** False belief that one is being harassed, cheated, or persecuted.
  - **Delusion of grandeur:** Exaggerated conception of one's own importance, power or identity. Individual believes that he is a great person with extra ordinary power, e.g. 'I have godly power and can predict things'
  - **Delusion of reference:** False belief that the behavior of others or happenings in the environment has a special reference to him/her.
  - **Delusion of infidelity:** Pathological jealousy that one's lover/partner is unfaithful.
  - **Delusion of guilt (Delusion of sin or self-accusation):** False feeling of guilt (Individual believes that he has done some unforgivable mistakes, but actually it is baseless).
  - **Somatic delusion:** False fixed belief involving functioning of one's body, e.g. individual may say that his heart is not beating.
  - **Nihilistic delusion:** False feeling that self, others or the world is nonexistent or feel as ending of all material possessions.
  - **Erotomania:** Delusional belief, more common in women, that a man who is not close to her (especially an eminent person) is deeply in love with her (Clerambault's syndrome).
  - **Hypochondriacal delusion:** Excessive fear of, or preoccupation with a serious illness, despite medical testing and reassurance, e.g. individual says that he is suffering from AIDS.
  - **Delusion of poverty:** Strong false belief that he is financially incapacitated, e.g. individual believe that his property and belongings had lost and he is poor and is not able to survive. But actually it is not the situation.
  - **Bizarre delusion:** A delusion that is very strange and completely impossible.

- **Mood-congruent delusion:** Any delusion with its content consistent with the sufferer's emotional state (either a depressive or manic state).

Disorders in the Possession of Thought (Thought Alienation Process)

- **Thought insertion:** Individual feels that thoughts are being inserted in him/her by others or by an external force.
- **Thought withdrawal:** Individual feels that thoughts are being taken away from his mind and he cannot think anymore.
- **Thought diffusion:** Individual feels that his thoughts are accessible to others as it escapes from his mind. In severe form it leads to thought broadcasting, where individual feels that his thoughts are being read aloud, or being broadcasted in radio or TV.

Table 5.4: Disorders of thought

A. Disturbance in the form and flow of thought	B. Disturbance in continuity of thought	C. Disturbance in the content of thought	D. Disturbance in the possession of thought.
- Psychomotor retardation - Thought blocking - Pressure of speech - Flight of ideas	- Circumstan-tiality - Tangentiality - Perseveration - Stereotype speech - Loosening of association - Incoherence - Word salad - Verbigeration - Clang association - Echolalia - Palilalia - Neologism	- Overvalued ideas - Fantasy - Idea of reference - Obsession - Phobia - Delusions	- Thought insertion - Thought withdrawal - Thought diffusion/ Thought broad-casting

Disorders of Speech

Communication problems occur from thought disorders, as thought is expressed in speech. Many of the thought and speech disorders are overlapping.

- **Pressure of speech:** Spontaneous rapid speech with increased amount, and difficult to interrupt.
- **Poverty of speech:** Reduction in amount and content of speech, with answering in one or two words.

- **Stuttering:** It is a disorder with repetition and prolongation of sound or word, that lead to impairment in fluency of speech, it is also called stammering.
- **Cluttering:** Speech characterized by erratic order with rapid jerky spurts, and is difficult to understand.

Disorders of Perception

Perception is the process of understanding the environmental stimuli received through sense organs. Disorders of perception mainly include Illusions and Hallucinations:

- **Illusions:** These are perceptual distortions with misinterpretation of the sensory stimulus.
- **Hallucinations:** It simply means imaginary perception. Sensory perception occurs in the absence of a corresponding real sensory stimulus. Hallucinations can occur in any sensory modality. Based on this, hallucinations are of different types as:
  - *Auditory hallucination:* Hearing sounds or speech in the absence of real auditory stimulus. Auditory hallucination can be of different types as:
    - **Audible thoughts:** Individual hears his own thoughts aloud. It is also known as 'thought echo'.
    - **Second person hallucination:** Individual hears the speech in second person as 'you', and speech involve 'the voice' and the individual.
    - **Third person hallucination:** Individual hears conversation about himself or herself, between two or more persons or parties.
    - **Command hallucinations:** These are frightening types of orders or commands, such as 'kill him with that knife.'
  - *Visual hallucinations:* Seeing things or persons in the absence of real external stimulus, e.g. seeing God or Goddess
  - *Olfactory hallucination:* Experience of smell in the absence of real stimulus, e.g. individual experience the smell of poison in food.
  - *Gustatory hallucination:* Experience of some taste in the absence of real stimulus.
  - *Tactile/Haptic hallucination:* Experience of touch sensation in the absence of real stimulus, e.g. individual experiences crawling sensation of insects over his body.
- Kinesthetic hallucination is the hallucination involving the sense of bodily movements.

  Olfactory and gustatory hallucinations are common in organic mental disorders. Tactile hallucination as feeling of bugs, crawling over the skin (Formication) as in case of alcohol withdrawal, and cocaine intoxication.

- **Depersonalization:** It is a perceptual disorder in which self appears as unreal to the individual.
- **Derealization:** Perceptual disorder in which the world appears to be unreal to the individual.

Disturbance in Emotions

Emotion: A complex subjective feeling state with psychic, somatic or physiological and behavioral components that is related to affect the mood.

Mood: It is the subjective, pervasive feeling tone that sustains for lengthy period.

Affect: It is the outward objective, but short lived experience at a given time.

Abnormal presence of emotions (as fear, anxiety, angry, sadness) can occur in mental illness. Sometimes abnormality can occur in depth and duration.

- **Blunted affect:** It is a disturbance in affect manifested by a severe reduction in the intensity of expression of feeling tone (greatly diminished emotional response).
- **Restricted or constricted affect:** There will be reduction in intensity of feeling tone, but less severe than blunted affect.
- **Flattened affect:** Absence or near absence of any signs of affective expression—patient presents with monotonous voice and immobile face. Absence of affect is called apathy. Seen in schizophrenia.
- **Elevated mood:** Expression of confidence and enjoyment with a more cheerful, which is more than normal; but not necessarily pathological.
- **Expansive mood:** Expression of one's feelings, with an overestimation of one's own importance.
- **Anhedonia:** Loss of interest in/withdrawal from all regular and pleasurable activities (Inability to experience pleasure). It is seen in depression and in schizophrenia, as its negative symptom.
- **Alexithymia:** It is the inability or difficulty in describing one's emotions or unable of being aware of one's emotions or mood.
- **Inappropriate affect:** Disharmony between the emotional feeling tone and the idea, thought or speech accompanying it.
- **Incongruent affect:** The expressed feelings are not congruent to the thought content. It is common in schizophrenia.
- **Labile affect:** Rapidly fluctuating emotional feeling tone, unrelated to external stimuli.

- **Ambivalence:** Coexistence of two opposing feelings or attitude towards person, idea or object.
- **Euphoria:** Increased sense of psychological well-being and happiness not associated with ongoing events.
- **Elation:** Moderate elevation of mood with increased psychomotor activity.
- **Exaltation:** Intense elevation of mood with delusion of grandeur.
- **Ecstasy:** Severe elevation of mood and intense blissfulness (seen in delirious mania).

Disorders of Consciousness

Consciousness is the state of awareness of self and the environment and the individual will be alert.

Disorders of Consciousness may occur in different forms as:

- **Confusion:** Inability to think clearly
- **Clouding of consciousness:** State with diminished alertness
- **Drowsiness:** State in which, the individual is awake, but looks and feels sleepy.
- **Stupor:** It is a diminished state of consciousness, where the individual remains unresponsive, immobile and mute, but eyes remain open and respiratory movements are there, but not aware of the surroundings.
- **Delirium:** Temporary state of clouding of consciousness, with restlessness, illusion, hallucination and apprehension.
- **Coma:** State of deep unconsciousness.
- **Fugue:** It is a state with mistaken identity and individual tends to wander away from normal surroundings.
- **Dissociation:** It is reversible and temporary alteration in consciousness and identity.

Disorders of Attention and Concentration

- Attention is the process of focusing consciousness on a particular object or idea.
- Concentration is the persistence of attention to the same stimuli. In mental illness, there will be some changes in these processes.
- **Distraction:** It is the problem of attention, where attention rapidly shifts from one thing to another and shows difficulty to sustain concentration.

Disorders of Orientation

Orientation is one's continuous awareness of person, place and time in relation to self and surroundings.

Orientation is affected in organic mental disorders.

- Disorientation to time occurs first, then place and person.
- Disorientation to one's own identity also can occur, especially with advanced age.

Disorders of Memory

- **Hypermnesia:** Unusually detailed and vivid memory is called hypermnesia.
- **Amnesia:** It is the loss of memory or inability to recall the stored information.
  It is usually organic in nature and can occur as:
  - *Retrograde amnesia:* Amnesia related to already existing memory or loss of memory that existed prior to a traumatic event or prior to a point of time.
  - *Anterograde amnesia:* Inability to form new memory or amnesia for events that occur after a trauma or a period of time.
- **Paramnesia**: Retrospective falsification or distortion of memory is called paramnesia.
  - *Confabulation:* Unintentional filling of memory gaps with fantasy or imagination. It is considered as a common type of paramnesia.
  - *Deja vu:* It is a problem with memory in which a new situation is felt as the repetition of previous one that has already seen, e.g. while visiting a temple for the first time, individual feels familiarity as he/she had visited there earlier.
  - *Jamais vu:* It is the feeling of temporary unfamiliarity with an already experienced or known situation, e.g. individual feels unfamiliarity to the place where he/she lives for the past five years.

Disturbance in Intelligence

Intelligence is the ability to think logically and to deal effectively with the environment, by relating it with previous knowledge and experience.

Disturbance in Intelligence also includes some problems in general knowledge, application of arithmetic abilities, reading and writing abilities and abstract thinking which involve concept formation. Inappropriate or concrete response indicates schizophrenia.

Disturbance in Judgment

Judgment is one's ability to assess accurately and to act appropriately to a situation. Normal, appropriate judgment needs correct perception, evaluation and ability for right conclusion/decision.

Judgment is usually impaired in many psychiatric problems as anxiety states, intoxication and in psychotic disorders, especially in schizophrenia.

Insight

Insight is the ability to understand self. In psychiatric assessment insight means the degree of awareness regarding one's illness. Insight can be graded in a six point scale.

Grading of Insight

I. Complete denial of illness.
II. Slight awareness of being sick, at the same time denies it.
III. Awareness of being sick, but it is attributed to external or physical factors.
IV. Awareness of being sick due to something unknown in him/her.
V. Intellectual insight—awareness of being sick—problems in social adjustment, irrational thoughts and feelings—but does not apply this knowledge to present or future.
VI. True emotional insight—individual is aware of illness and apply this knowledge for basic changes in future behavior.

Physical Manifestations of Mental Illness

Some physical manifestations can also occur along with the problems in higher mental functions. They are:

- **Disturbance in volition:**
  - **Volition** is the willful initiation and control of one's own behavior. Usually people willfully initiate and control their behavior.
  - **Avolition:** Absence of willful initiation and control of behavior. It is usually seen along with immobility, mutism, and stupor in Schizophrenia.
- **Alteration in biological functioning:** Many people report lack of sleep or increased sleep, decrease or increase of appetite in the early stage of disorders.

Sleep Problems

- **Insomnia:** It is the difficulty in initiation or maintenance of sleep. Usually seen in mania. This can occur as early, late and middle insomnia.
- **Reversal of sleep-wake pattern:** Here the rhythm of sleep is reversed (Individual sleeps during daytime and will be awake during night). It is usually associated with organic conditions like dementia or delirium.
- **Narcolepsy:** Sudden attack of irresistible pattern of sleep, seen in cataplexy (Sudden attack of severe generalized muscle weakness leading to physical collapse in an alert state).

- **Hypersomnia:** Increased sleep is also considered as abnormal. Individual sleeps excessively during daytime.
- **Somnolence:** It is a sleep disturbance, characterized by abnormal drowsiness during day time/excess day time sleep.
- **Somnambulism:** Sleep walking.
- **Somniloquy:** Speaking in sleep.

Appetite Changes

It is usually observed in many cases, but in most cases patients are not reporting it. But we should ask about the details of eating pattern of patient from the relative/informant.

- **Increased appetite:** It is seen in mania and in endocrine problems like hyperthyroidism. During the initial stage of mania, patient eats voraciously. But as the hyperactivity increases, it will not be easy for them to sit still. Overeating may also be seen in atypical depression and bulimic syndrome.
- **Decreased appetite:** Marked decrease in appetite is seen in depression/anxiety and in anorexia nervosa.
- **Pica:** Eating non edible things like mud, chalk piece, hair, etc.
  In schizophrenia, any of this can occur.

Change in Sexual Desire

This is reported in mental illness as either increased or decreased.

- Increased sexual desire (hypersexuality) may occur in mania, and in neuro problems like cerebral lesions.
- Sexual desire is decreased in anxiety, depression, drug abuse and in some endocrine problems.

Loss of libido, erectile dysfunctions, ejaculatory disturbances and pain are seen in psychosexual disorders.

CONCLUSION

In this chapter the etiology and clinical features of mental disorders were explained along brief review of structure and functions of brain. The role of different neurotransmitters and their correlation with mental disorders will enable better understanding of psychopathology. Knowledge about signs and symptoms of mental illness will be useful in assessment and provision of care.

BIBLIOGRAPHY

1. Ahuja N. A Short Textbook of Psychiatry (Seventh edition). New Delhi: Jaypee Brothers Medicl Publishers (P) Ltd, 2011.

2. Fontaine KL. Mental Health Nursing (Fifth edition). New Delhi: Pearson Education, 2009.
3. Kapoor B. Textbook of Psychiatric Nursing. Delhi: Kumar Publishing House, 2014.
4. Lalitha K. Mental Health and Psychiatric Nursing an Indian Perspective. Bangaluru: VMG Book House, 2008.
5. Sadock BJ, Sadock VA, Ruiz P. Kaplan and Sadock's Synopsis of Psychiatry: Behavioral Sciences/Clinical Psychiatry (Ninth edition). Philadelphia: Wolters Kluwer, 2009.
6. Townsend CM. Psychiatric Mental Health Nursing: Concepts of Care in Evidence-Based Practice (7th Edition). Philadelphia: FA Davis Company, 2012.

CHAPTER 6 Biopsychosocial Therapies

INTRODUCTION

In the early periods due to the misconceptions of mental illness, lot of primitive methods like trephining was used as treatment measures. Treatment approach of an illness varies with its underlying etiology and clinical features. Due to the lack of definite etiology, the treatment of mental disorders was a challenge in the early periods. But with the invention of chlorpromazine in 1952, there was marked change in the management of these disorders. Psychosocial therapies are also equally important in the management of mental illness due to the psychosocial aspects in the etiology.

Therapies in psychiatric problems can be broadly divided as:

- Biological therapies
- Psychosocial therapy

Drug therapy and somatic therapy like electroconvulsive therapy (ECT) can be considered as biological therapies. These are used in acute phase and drugs are continued as maintenance therapy.

Psychosocial therapies include different psychotherapies and behavior therapies. These are used when acute phase is settled and also can be used as preventive approach.

PSYCHOPHARMACOLOGY

Psychopharmacology is the study of drugs that have effect on thoughts, emotions and behavior, that are used to treat psychiatric disorders.

Psychotropic Drugs

The drugs that influence the synaptic transmission in brain and cause changes in the physiological and psychological functions, emotions and behavior. They can make significant effects on higher mental functions.

Neurotransmission

Neurotransmitters are the chemical messengers that enables neurotransmission in the synapse. They are synthesized by enzymes from certain dietary amino acids.

Neurotransmitters are stored in axon terminals of presynaptic neuron. As electrical impulses travels through neuron, it stimulates the release of neurotransmitters into the synaptic cleft which causes nerve impulse transmission.

After neurotransmission, they are either reabsorbed (reuptaken), and stored in presynaptic neuron for later use, or it may be metabolized by enzyme like monoamine oxidase and cholinesterase.

Effects of Psychotropic Drugs on Neurotransmission

Psychotropic drugs influence behavior by altering the activity of neurotransmitters. Drugs may decrease or increase the amount or effect of neurotransmitters by different means:

- **Release effect:** These drugs release more neurotransmitters into synapse and increases the impulse transmission.
- **Blockade effect:** Drugs will prevent the neurotransmitters from binding with postsynaptic receptors through its blockade action.
- **Receptor sensitivity changes:** Drugs make the receptors more or less responsive to the neurotransmitters and influence neurotransmission.
- **Blockage of reuptake:** Drugs will hinder the re-absorption of neurotransmitters to presynaptic cells and thus it is retained in the synapse and prolongs its action.
- **Interference with storage:** Some drugs act by interfering with the storage of neurotransmitters and thus it is more or less released and influence impulse transmission.
- **Precursor chain interference:** Drugs may interfere the process of synthesis of neurotransmitter from its precursor, so the excess production of neurotransmitters is decreased and thus reduce impulse transmission.

Special Considerations in the Administration of Psychotropic Drugs

- **Therapeutic index of drug:** It is a relative measure of the safety and toxicity of a drug. Low therapeutic index means the difference between the amount of drug needed to achieve the desired effect and amount that would cause toxic effects has narrow range, e.g. Lithium has low therapeutic index and requires frequent blood level checks and careful monitoring of drug. But serenace has high therapeutic index, so can be prescribed in a wide range of dose.
- **Old age:** In old age, hepatic and renal clearance of drugs is decreased. So start with low dose and go slow while increasing the dose. They are on multiple drugs for different illness. So be careful against drug interaction.
- **Children:** In case of children, correct dose must be given, by considering body weight, body size. Close observation is essential.

- Pregnant/lactating women need special consideration because some of these drugs have teratogenic effects.
- Age, gender, and race also can affect the therapeutic effect of specific drug.
- Some patients become less responsive to same dose of specific drug over time, and it is called tolerance.
- Drug co-administration may be beneficial or it may cause risk of increase side effects due to drug interaction.

Classification of Psychotropic Drugs

Psychotropic drugs are classified as follows, based on their indications:
- Antipsychotics
- Antidepressants
- Mood stabilizing drugs
- Antianxiety and hypnosedatives
- Antiparkinsonian drugs.

ANTIPSYCHOTIC DRUGS

Definition

Psychotropic drugs which are used in the treatment of psychotic disorders and psychotic symptoms are called antipsychotics.

These are the D2 receptor blockers (dopamine receptor blockers)—used in the treatment of psychosis, for relief of psychotic symptoms.

Other names for this group are neuroleptics or ataractics or major tranquilizers or antischizophrenics.

Indications

- **Organic psychiatric disorders:**
  - Delirium
  - Dementia
  - Delirium tremens
  - Substance induced psychosis.
- **Non-organic (functional psychiatric disorders):**
  - Acute psychosis
  - Schizophrenia
  - Schizoaffective disorders
  - Delusional disorders
  - Mania with psychotic symptoms
  - Depression with psychotic symptoms
  - Childhood psychiatric disorders (only after 5 years).
- **Medical disorders:**
  - Huntington's chorea
  - Tic disorders.

Target Symptoms of Antipsychotics

Both typical and atypical antipsychotics are used for treatment of:

- Psychotic symptoms—as delusion and hallucinations (all sensory type).
- Disorganization of speech and behavior.
- Positive formal thought disorders (incoherence, derailment, illogicity).
- Bizarre behavior (catatonic motor behavior, disorders of movement, deterioration of social behavior).

Contraindications of Antipsychotics

- Children below three years
- Severe depression
- Hypersensitivity
- Parkinsonism
- Glaucoma
- Severe hepatic or renal disease
- Severe hypertension
- Patients with bone marrow depression.

Special precaution is needed in patients with Parkinson's disease, pregnancy, epilepsy.

Classification of Antipsychotics (Table 6.1)

Antipsychotics are broadly categorized as:

- Typical antipsychotics
- Aytpical antipsychotics

Table 6.1: Classification of antipsychotics

Name of drug	*Dosage (mg/day)*	
• Typical antipsychotics		
– Chlorpromazine	300–1000	50–1000 mg IM
– Fluphenazine	2–20	
– Haloperidol	5–30	5–10 mg IM
– Loxapine	25–250	
– Pimozide	4–20	
– Prochlorperazine	45–150	
– Thioridazine	300–600	
– Trifluoperazine	15–50	
• Atypical antipsychotics		
– Clozapine	50–900	
– Olanzapine	5–20	
– Quetiapine	150–750	
– Risperidone	2–8	
– Ziprasidone	40–160	
– Aripiprazole	5–30	

Typical Antipsychotics or Conventional Antipsychotics or First Generation Antipsyhotics

These drugs were developed in 1950s. Chlorpromazine was the first antipsychotic used in treatment of mental disorders. Haloperidol is another potent drug used in the treatment of psychotic symptoms in severe cases (presence of severe side effects of these drugs led to the invention of atypical antipsychotics or second generation drugs).

Mechanism of Action of Typical Antipsychotics

Typical antipsychotics mainly act by its antidopaminergic activity. These drugs block D2 receptors in the mesolimbic and mesocortical systems which are concerned with emotional reactions and thus control psychotic features.

Along with this desired effect, the drug acts on some other areas of brain and causes the following side effects:

- Extrapyramidal symptoms (EPS) is a major side effect, caused by anti-dopaminergic action on basal ganglia/nigrostriatal system.
- Hyperprolactinemia due to blockade of tuberoinfundibular system.
- Sedation due to alpha-adrenergic blockade/histaminergic action (more with chlorpromazine and thioridazine).
- Orally administered drug is absorbed from gastrointestinal tract and brain concentration is more than plasma concentration. Drugs get metabolized in liver, excreted through the kidneys. They easily enter areas with good blood supply (brain, lung, kidney and fetus). Drug is not dialyzable also.

Atypical Antipsychotics

These are weaker dopamine receptor antagonists that act by selective limbic dopamine blockade action—D4 receptor blockade or a combination of potent antagonist of 5HT2 (serotonin type 2) and weak D2 antagonistic (antiserotonergic and selective dopamine blockade action). So these drugs do not have side effects like tardive dyskinesia, neuroleptic malignant syndrome and less chance for EPS.

Specific Situations where Atypical Antipsychotics are Preferred

- Negative symptoms of schizophrenia
  - Affective flattening
  - Alogia
  - Avolition/Apathy
  - Anhedonia
  - Asociality
  - Attentional impairment
- Mood symptoms
- Cognitive impairment
- Difficulty with socialization.

Advantages of Atypical Antipsychotics

- Atypical antipsychotics are effective against both positive and negative symptoms of schizophrenia.
- It rarely causes extrapyramidal symptoms.
- Used to treat—mood symptoms, hostility, violence, suicidal behavior, asociality and cognitive impairment.

Mechanism of Action of Atypical Antipsychotics

They exert blocking effects at D2 and Serotonin 2 postsynaptic receptor (serotonin-dopamine antagonist). They have antiserotonergic, anti-adrenergic and antihistaminergic actions.

Clozapine was the first new generation antipsychotic, which was rediscovered in 1988 and effectively used for treatment of refractory schizophrenia.

Specific Side Effects of Atypical Antipsychotics

- Obesity—due to histamine antagonism which increases appetite.
- Diabetes mellitus
- Metabolic syndrome which includes:
  - Obesity
  - Increased blood pressure
  - Increased blood sugar
  - Increased cholesterol with > 150 mg TG.

Side Effects of Antipsychotics (General)

- Extrapyramidal symptoms (EPS)
- Other central nervous system (CNS) side effects
- Autonomic side effects
- Metabolic and endocrine side effect
- Allergic side effects
- Cardiac side effects
- Ocular side effects
- Dermatological side effects.

Extrapyramidal Side Effects

Serious neurologic symptoms that occur due to blockade of D2 receptors in the midbrain part of brain stem. This includes:

- Neuroleptic induced parkinsonism
- Akathisia
- Acute dystonia
- Tardive dyskinesia
- Neuroleptic malignant syndrome (NMS).

Neuroleptic-induced Parkinsonism

It is more with typical antipsychotics. Parkinsonian features like:

- Rigidity and Bradykinesia or Akinesia
- Tremors (pill rolling tremors)
- Stooped stiff posture
- Drooling
- Shuffling gait and Ataxia.

(Parkinsonian side effects are less with atypical antipsychotics and maximum with haloperidol which is a typical antipsychotic).

Management—stop the drug.

Administer anticholinergics or antiparkinsonian drugs.

Akathisia (Motor Restlessness)

Patient paces constantly—'walking in place' or moves legs while sitting. There is a subjective feeling of muscular discomfort that leads to agitation, restlessness, and dysphoria (akathisia is maximum with haloperidol and minimum with clozapine and quetiapine).

Management—stop drug

Administer propranolol, benzodiazepines or clonidine.

Acute Dystonia

It is the bizarre painful muscle spasm or contractions which involve head, jaw, tongue and neck muscles. Along with this, upward lateral movement of eye, with turning of head to one side may occur and is called oculogyric crisis. Sometime trunk and lower extremities or entire body spasm may occur and may lead to opisthotonus.

Management—stop drug.

Administer anticholinergics or benzodiazepine.

Phenergan is the most commonly used drug and is usually prescribed along with haloperidol to prevent dystonia.

Tardive Dyskinesia

It is the late onset of orofacial dyskinesia. Features are abnormal, irregular choreoathetoid movement of muscles of head, limbs, and trunk, characterized by chewing, sucking, grimacing and perioral movements. This occurs due to D2 receptor supersensitivity. This side effect is minimum with clozapine. There is no effective treatment for tardive dyskinesia. Prevention is better.

Neuroleptic Malignant Syndrome (NMS)

Rapid onset of severe motor, mental and autonomic symptoms occur in 24–72 hrs of administration of antipsychotics.

- **Motor symptoms:** Generalized muscular hypertonicity that leads to stiffness of muscles of throat and chest leading to dysphagia, and dyspnea.
- **Mental symptoms:** Akinetic mutism, stupor or alteration in consciousness.
- **Autonomic nervous system side effects:** Hyperpyrexia, unstable blood pressure, tachycardia, excess sweating and salivation, urinary incontinence.

Blood test will show increased creatine phosphokinase (CPK) and increased white blood cell count.

Secondary Features or Complications of NMS: Pneumonia, thromboembolism, cardiovascular collapse and renal failure.

Management: Bromocriptine, dantrolene, baclofen are some of the drugs used. Along with this, general supportive care with symptomatic management.

Other CNS Side Effects

- Dizziness—due to alpha adrenergic blockade.
- Seizures—due to decrease in seizure threshold.
- Sedation and weight gain—due to histaminergic blockade.
- Depression or pseudodepression—due to decreased catecholamine which is treated with antidepressants and rarely treated with electroconvulsive therapy.

Other Side Effects

- **Autonomic side effects:**
  - Dry mouth
  - Constipation
  - Urinary retention (rule out benign prostatic hypertrophy)
  - Orthostatic hypotension due to alpha-1 adrenergic blockade effect
  - Mydriasis
  - Impotence or impaired ejaculation.
- **Metabolic and endocrine side effects:**
  - Weight gain
  - Diabetes
  - Galactorrhea with or without amenorrhea.
- **Allergic side effects:**
  - Cholestatic jaundice
  - Agranulocytosis (maximum with clozapine).
- **Cardiac side effects:**
  - Electrocardiogram (ECG) changes
  - Very rarely ventricular fibrillation and death.

- **Ocular side effects:**
  - Blurring of vision
  - Pigmentary retinopathy
  - Granular deposits in cornea and lens due to photosensitivity.
- **Dermatological side effects:**
  - Photosensitivity reaction
  - Contact dermatitis
  - Blue gray metallic discoloration.
- **Gastrointestinal side effects:**
  - Anorexia, nausea, vomiting
  - Obstructive jaundice (malaise, nausea, pruritus and jaundice).

Nurse's Responsibilities while Caring Patients Receiving Antipsychotics

In mental health nursing, apart from the general considerations in medicine administration, nurse must make sure that patient has swallowed the medications, because patient may deny his illness and the need for medication. Nurses must have good knowledge about psychopharmacology—the action, side effects and their management. Patient may not be reporting the side effects or the desired effect, so it is the nurse's responsibility to observe for both and to report it to the doctor or to manage the side effects with appropriate action.

Nurses must observe the behavior pattern, and must assess the thought process, speech, perception and cognitive functions.

Nurse must observe for extrapyramidal side effects, report it to the doctor and manage it with specific medications as per order.

Nursing Management of Side Effects of Antipsychotics

Autonomic side effects or anticholinergic side effects

- **Dry mouth:** Give frequent oral sips of fluid and increase fluid intake, also ensure good oral hygiene.
- **Constipation:** Increase fluid intake and encourage roughage containing foods. Motivate and engage the client in physical activities.
- **Urinary retention:** Monitor fluid intake and output. Ask for any difficulty in urination and ask about benign prostatic hypertrophy and report it.
- **Blurring of vision:** Mydriasis and vision problems usually settle by few weeks. Advise client not to drive vehicles and to be more careful in all activities, especially while walking to prevent accidents.
- **Orthostatic hypotension:** Monitor blood pressure in standing and lying position and report, if there is any marked variation. Ambulation must be done slowly and carefully to prevent falls. Advise the client to prevent sudden change of position.

- **Sedation:** It is another side effect. So advise the patient not to drive vehicles or to handle heavy machinery. Usually these drugs are administered at bed time.
- **Sexual problems:** Impotence or problems with ejaculation must be reported to the doctor, so that dose may be adjusted.

Metabolic or endocrine side effects

- Do a baseline assessment of bodyweight and monitor weight at least twice a week.
- Encourage low calorie diet and physical exercise. Advise to avoid fried foods and sweet items.
- Metabolic syndrome which includes obesity, diabetes mellitus, hypertension, hypercholesterolemia are common with atypical antipsychotics. So monitor blood sugar, blood pressure and serum cholesterol and educate about prevention of these problems.

Galactorrhea is a common side effect with typical antipsychotics, seen in females. Males may present with gynecomastia. So these side effects must be identified early with assessment and interview.

Allergic Side Effects

Observe for signs and symptoms of cholestatic jaundice (pruritus, jaundice, pale stool and dark urine).

Observe for skin rashes as it can occur with both typical and atypical antipsychotics.

Agranulocytosis is common with typical antipsychotics and with clozapine, which is an atypical one. So do a baseline assessment of total and differential count of blood cells before starting clozapine and monitor the white blood cells (WBC) count during therapy. Observe this patient for sore throat or frequent respiratory infections and treat it early.

Monitor the blood count for patients receiving clozapine because agranulocytosis is a major side effect of it. WBC must be at least 3500/ mm^3, and must be checked biweekly in the initial period and then checked in every 4 weeks. After discontinuing the medication WBC count must be checked for 4 weeks more.

Cardiac Side Effects

ECG changes especially prolongation of QT interval can occur. So before starting antipsychotics, a baseline ECG must be taken.

Very rarely arrhythmias can occur. Check pulse rate for full minute. Monitor ECG in every 3–6 months or as required.

Ocular Side Effects

Photosensitivity can occur with both the type of antipsychotics. Advise the client to wear protective sunglass when they go outside. If granular deposits in cornea occur, the drug must be changed.

Ophthalmic check up is essential in 3–6 months, or if the patient develops any visual problems. This will help in identifying and treating the pigmentary retinopathy, and granular deposits in cornea or lens.

Dermatological Side Effects

Photosensitivity can occur in skin also. Instruct the client to wear full sleeve clothes and sun block lotions while going out or work in sunlight.

Drug Adherence or Drug Compliance and Nurse's Role

Drug compliance in patients receiving antipsychotics is very difficult due to many reasons and poor treatment adherence leads to relapses. Nurse must identify the reason for noncompliance and must educate and give guidance to the caregivers about the need of regular treatment and follow up (Table 6.2).

Psychoeducation

Nurse must educate the caregivers about the specific observations, side effects and its management as mentioned in the nursing management. Emphasize the need of regular treatment and follow up in the prevention of relapse.

Table 6.2: Factors leading to noncompliance

- Distressing side effects
- Slow onset of desired effects
- Need for several doses per day or due to the complexity of therapy
- Most of the drugs are orally administered, but patient may deny the need for treatment due to lack of insight
- Lack of knowledge regarding illness, treatment and side effects
- Due to the stigma of mental disorder
- Poor social support
- Lack of awareness on availability of treatments and other services
- Presence of persecutory delusion and hopelessness.

Since irregular treatment leads to relapse, long acting antipsychotics are preferred in patients who are with poor drug compliance. Antipsychotic depot preparations are given intramuscularly in every 2–4 weeks. Injections must be given as deep intramuscular (IM), otherwise tissue irritation can occur. This group of drugs are useful in patients.

Commonly used depot preparations are:

- Fluphenazine decanoate 12.5–100 mg IM every 2–4 weeks or 25 mg IM every 2 weeks.
- Flupenthixol decanoate 20–300 mg IM every 2–4 weeks.
- Risperidone consta 25–50 mg IM every 2 weeks.

ANTIDEPRESSANTS

These are the specific group of drugs used in the treatment of depressive illness. They are also known as mood elevators or thymoleptics. In mood disorders, basic etiology is the dysregulation of serotonin, norepinephrine and other neurotransmitters. Antidepressant improve neurotransmission through different actions:

- By blocking the reuptake of neurotransmitters in the presynaptic neuron.
- By inhibiting the metabolism and subsequent deactivation of specific neurotransmitters.
- By affecting the activity of postsynaptic receptors.
- They enhance the communication in the brain structures that are responsible for mood and emotion and anxiety disorders.

Antidepressants take several weeks to show clinical improvements or its effect on mood, because the receptors take several weeks to return to their normal synaptic activity.

Indications for Antidepressants

- **Depression:**
  - Acute depression
  - Depression with psychotic features
  - Dysthymia
  - Secondary depression
  - Abnormal grief reaction
  - Bipolar depression
  - Atypical depression.
- **Childhood psychiatric disorders:**
  - Enuresis
  - Separation anxiety disorder
  - Somnambulism
  - School phobia.
- **Other psychiatric disorders:**
  - Panic attack
  - Generalized anxiety disorder
  - Obsessive-compulsive disorder with depression
  - Eating disorders
  - Borderline personality disorder
  - Post-traumatic stress disorder
  - Agoraphobia and social phobia.
- **Medical disorders:**
  - Chronic pain
  - Migraine
  - Peptic ulcer disease.

Target Symptoms for Use of Antidepressants

- Suicidal thoughts
- Middle and terminal insomnia
- Appetite disturbances
- Anxiety disorders
- Somatic complaints with agitation
- Motor retardation with dysphoric mood.

Contraindications/Specific Precautions in Antidepressant Therapy

Patients with:

- Cardiovascular disease due to risk of arrhythmia
- Severe psychotic symptoms
- Liver disease
- Seizure.

Classification of Antidepressants

Classification of antidepressants is shown in Table 6.3.

Table 6.3: Classification of antidepressants

Name of antidepressants	*Dosage (mg/day)*
Cyclic Antidepressants	
• **Tricyclic Antidepressants**	
– Amitriptyline	75–300
– Clomipramine	75–250
– Imipramine	75–300
– Doxepin	75–300
– Desipramine	75–300
– Nortriptyline	75–100
• **Tetracyclic Antidepressants**	
– Amoxapine	150–400
– Mianserin	30–120
– Maprotiline	75–225
Selective Serotonin Reuptake Inhibitor (SSRI)	
• Fluoxetine	10–60
• Paroxetine	10–40
• Fluvoxamine	50–300
• Sertraline	50–200
• Citalopram	10–40
Serotonin Norepinephrine Reuptake Inhibitor (SNRI)	
• Venlafaxine	75–375
• Duloxetine	60
Norepinephrine Dopamine Reuptake Inhibitor (NDRI)	
• Bupropion	150–450
Monoamine Oxidase Inhibitors (MAOIs)	
• Selegiline	5–10

Pharmacokinetics

Oral tricyclic antidepressants (TCA) are highly anticholinergic in action, they delay gastric emptying by slowing the gastrointestinal mobility, and are not absorbed well. With regular administration of TCA, a steady blood level is attained by the end of 2 weeks or in 2–3 weeks. Antidepressants increase the catecholamine levels in brain.

Tricyclic antidepressants also known as monoamine reuptake inhibitors. They act by blocking the reuptake of norepinephrine, serotonin and/or dopamine at the nerve terminals. This causes increase in these neurotransmitters at the receptor site. Along with this there is down regulation of beta adrenergic receptors. But SSRI are well absorbed in gastrointestinal tract. They are highly protein bound and accumulates in vascular areas. These drugs are not dialyzable.

SSRI inhibit the reuptake of serotonin selectively and increase its availability at the receptor site.

Monoamine oxidase inhibitors (MAO inhibitors) act by inhibiting the monoamine oxidase which oxidize or degrade the catecholamines after its reuptake. This will lead to increase in the bioavailability of norepinephrine and/or serotonin at the receptor site. MAO inhibitors maintain a steady blood level by 5–10 days.

Antidepressants must be continued for six to twelve months, even after the remission of symptoms in the first episode of depression and continued for longer duration in the subsequent episodes.

Side Effects of Antidepressants

Many of the side effects of antidepressants are similar to that of antipsychotics and are shown in Table 6.4.

Table 6.4: Side effects of antidepressants

- **Autonomic side effects:**
  - Dry mouth
  - Constipation
  - Urinary retention
  - Mydriasis
  - Aggravation of narrow angle glaucoma (due to muscarinic cholinergic blockade action)
  - Orthostatic hypotension (due to alpha adrenergic blockade action)
- **Central nervous system (CNS) side effects:**
  - Sedation and drowsiness (due to alpha adrenergic blockade action)
  - Jitteriness syndrome (due to adrenergic and serotonergic action)
  - Tremor and other extrapyramidal symptoms (EPS)
  - Withdrawal syndrome (due to dependence)
  - Seizures (as the drug decreases seizure threshold)
  - Aggravation of psychotic symptoms like delusions and hallucinations and precipitation of mania (due to sympathomimetic action).

Contd...

Contd...

- **Cardiovascular side effects:**
  - Tachycardia, Hypertension, Electrocardiogram (ECG) changes (arrhythmias)
- **Allergic side effects:**
  - Agranulocytosis, cholestatic jaundice, skin rashes (due to hypersensitivity)
- **Metabolic and endocrine side effects:**
  - Weight gain
- **Sexual side effects:**
  - Impotence, impaired ejaculation
- **Hypertensive crisis** in monoamine oxidase (MAO) inhibitor receiving patients (due to interaction with the tyramine in food).
- **Severe hepatic necrosis** (due to hypersensitive or toxic effect)

Nurse's Role in Antidepressant Therapy

- Accurate observation and recording must be done on side effects and desired effects of drugs.
- Risk for committing suicide is more in early periods of antidepressant therapy, as this drug will increase the energy level and will help the patient in implementing their suicide plans. So close observation is essential while caring these patients.
- Administer drug at bed time due to sedative effects, or as prescribed by the doctor.
- Increase fluid intake and give frequent sips of fluid or chewing gum to manage dryness of mouth.
- Increase fluid intake and encourage roughage containing foods. Encourage physical activity to prevent constipation.
- Assess fluid intake and output. Ask for difficulty in urination or history of benign prostatic hypertrophy.
- Ask for any vision problem. Advise ophthalmic check up in every two months, to identify glaucoma in its early stage.
- Advise the patient to avoid sudden change of position to avoid giddiness and falls due to orthostatic hypotension.
- Check blood pressure at regular interval as there is risk for hypertension also.
- Warn the patient not to drive vehicles, or to operate heavy mechines due to the risk of accidents from sedation.
- Closely observe for side effects like tremors, EPS or aggravation of psychotic symptoms.
- Take safety precautions against seizure, because these drugs decrease the seizure threshold.
- Take a baseline ECG and check blood pressure before starting antidepressants. Monitor BP and pulse rate and report if there is marked variation.

- Check blood count before starting antidepressants, because agranulocytosis can occur as a side effect. Observe whether the patient has sore throat, fever and fatigue, that indicate agranulocytosis and monitor the blood count.
- Observe for skin rashes and signs and symptoms of cholestatic jaundice.
- Check body weight before starting antidepressants, and monitor for obesity as it is a side effect.
- If patient complaints of sexual dysfunctions, report to the doctor and stop the medication.
- Observe the patient for development of features of mania, and report it promptly.
- Patients receiving MAO inhibitors must be warned against tyramine containing foods (cheese, red wine, chicken liver), because it can cause hypertensive crisis. So nurse must educate patient and family and should observe for features like occipital headache or features of stroke.
- Do liver function tests before starting antidepressants.
- Interaction between MAO inhibitors and tricyclic antidepressants like imipramine can cause hyperpyrexia. So there must be a gap of one week between these drugs.
- Tricyclic antidepressants have dangerous cardiac side effects, and need monitoring of ECG. It is contraindicated in patients with cardiac conduction problems. Elderly people need only small dose and overdose may lead to death.
- Educate the patient and the caregiver about the side effects and its management, need for long-term treatment and regular follow up.
- Advise the caregiver to be supportive in stress situations.

MOOD STABILIZERS

These are the drugs that are effective in the treatment of mania and the mood swings in bipolar disorders. These drugs act as prophylactic agent and mood stabilizer. Commonly used mood stabilizers are:

- Lithium
- Sodium valproate
- Carbamazepine
- Oxcarbazepine.

Many of the atypical antipsychotics like Olanzapine, Quetiapine, Aripiprazole are used in the maintenance therapy of bipolar disorders.

Lithium

Lithium is being used in the treatment of mania in 1949, by John Cade. Lithium is known as antimanic agent or the drug of choice for mania. It is having mood stabilizing effect and prevent mood swings.

Indications

- Treatment of acute mania
- Prophylactic treatment of bipolar mood disorder.

Clinically Preferred in the Treatment

- Schizoaffective disorder
- Cyclothymia
- Acute depression
- Chronic alcoholism with depressive symptoms
- Cocaine dependence
- Impulsive aggression.

Mechanism of Action of Lithium

Though the exact mechanism is not known, it influences the action of many neurotransmitters. The following actions decrease the catecholamine activities and thus helps in managing mania:

- Lithium inhibits the release of catecholamines at the synapse.
- It increases the presynaptic reuptake and destruction of catecholamines like norepinephrine.
- It decreases the postsynaptic receptor sensitivity to serotonin 2 (5-HT2).
- Along with calcium and magnesium ion, lithium stabilizes the cell membrane.

For lithium there is a lag period of 7–10 days for the onset of action which is the time taken for achieving a steady level.

Lithium has very narrow therapeutic index, so it can easily cause lithium toxicity, which is fatal. Frequent monitoring of serum lithium will help in preventing lithium toxicity. Initially serum lithium is checked 2–3 times in a week because there is a lag period of 7–10 days before the onset of steady action.

Pharmacokinetics

Lithium is absorbed from gastrointestinal tract, and peak serum level is attained between 30 minutes to 3 hours. Absorption will be completed in 8 hours and maximum level occur in thyroid (so there is more chance for developing hypothyroidism).

Lithium is excreted by kidneys. As proximal reabsorption is influenced by sodium balance, sodium depletion will result in lithium toxicity.

Lithium has side effects at different systems in the body and there is more chance for lithium toxicity. So some investigations must be done before starting it, and also must be monitored at regular intervals.

Prelithium work up includes:

- Renal function test
- Thyroid function test

- ECG and cardiac work up
- Neurological assessment.

Once lithium is started, serum lithium must be monitored at regular intervals. Blood sample collection for lithium estimation must be done 12 hours after the last dose. If any adjustment in dose is done, serum lithium estimation must be done after 7 days of change in dose. Therapeutic level of lithium is 0.8–1.2 mEq/liter and prophylactic dose is 0.6–1.2 mEq/liter. If serum lithium is more than 2 mEq/liter, lithium toxicity occurs.

Lithium should not be stopped suddenly, it must be tapered and off. Lithium is available in two forms—lithium carbonate and lithium citrate. Lithium carbonate is commonly used and dose is 600–1200 mg in divided dose.

Side Effects of Lithium

Lithium has many side effects, and life-threatening, one is lithium intoxication [toxicity occurs if serum lithium is > 3.5 mEq/liter (Table 6.5)].

Table 6.5: Signs and symptoms of lithium toxicity

Lithium toxicity—signs and symptoms
• Coarse tremor of hands, muscle twitching, muscle weakness, ataxia, dysarthria
• Nausea and vomiting
• Impaired concentration and memory, confusion, lethargy
• Convulsions, hyperreflexia, nystagmus, coma
• Nephrotoxicity

Other Side Effects

- **Nervous system side effects:**
  - Tremor
  - Muscular weakness or fatigue
  - Cogwheel rigidity
  - Confusion, slurring of speech, tinnitus, blurring of vision
  - Seizures due to decrease of seizure threshold
  - Neurotoxicity leads to delirium, ataxia, involuntary movement, seizure and coma.
- **Renal side effects:**
  - Polyuria, polydypsia, nephrogenic diabetes insipidus, tubular changes and nephrotic syndrome.
- **Cardiovascular side effects:**
  - ECG changes T-wave depression
- **Endocrine side effects:**
  - Goiter, hypothyroidism, (abnormal thyroid function tests, weight gain and pedal edema)

- **Gastrointestinal side effects:**
  - Nausea, vomiting, diarrhea, abdominal pain, metallic taste in mouth.
- **Dermatological side effects:**
  - Acne, papular eruptions and exacerbation of psoriasis. Allergic reactions as itching or hair loss also can occur.
- **Side effects during pregnancy:**
  - Teratogenic effect (Ebstein anomaly—downward displacement of tricuspid valve in fetus).

Contraindications of lithium therapy are:

- Renal dysfunctions
- Cardiac diseases
- Blood dyscrasias
- First trimester of pregnancy and lactation
- Patients on diuretic therapy
- Patients with severe hypothyroidism need special precaution.

Patients receiving ACE inhibitors or angiotensin II receptor antagonists and NSAIDs (Non-steroidal anti-inflammatory drugs) need special precaution against toxicity especially if they are elderly.

Nurse's Responsibilities in Lithium Therapy

Apart from the general responsibilities, some specific care aspects in lithium therapy are:

- **Prelithium work up** should be done before starting lithium to find out any contraindication or special precaution.
- **Observe and report specific side effects** of lithium. Check serum lithium level and monitor for any symptoms of toxicity.
- **Intake-output chart** must be maintained to monitor renal functions and fluid balance must be maintained.
- **Record body weight** before starting lithium. This will help in assessing weight gain or fluid retention and ankle edema in renal problems.
- Observe and record body weight every week.
- **Increase fluid intake up to 3.0 liters** (if there is no fluid restriction), to balance the side effects like polydypsia, polyuria and to maintain fluid balance.
- **Do not restrict salt in the diet** of patients receiving lithium, because proxymal reabsorption of lithium is influenced by sodium level.
- Monitor renal function, thyroid function and serum electrolyte level as directed by doctor.
- Administer lithium along with foods to prevent metallic taste in mouth.

- Patient and caregiver must be warned against the repetition of dose if they have forgotten a dose. It is better to skip that dose, to prevent the risk of toxicity.
- Patient and family must be educated about prevention of dehydration and sodium depletion. If patient has fever, diarrhea, vomiting, excess sweating, or if the patient is on diuretics, special precaution is needed.
- Educate patient and family about the side effects of lithium and features of lithium toxicity, need for serum lithium estimation, regular follow up and specific observations and care in lithium therapy.
- Blood for serum lithium estimation should be collected 12 hours after the last dose of lithium.

Sodium Valproate

Sodium valproate is also used for prophylaxis of bipolar disorders and for migraine headache prophylaxis. Exact mechanism of action is not clear.

Indications

- **Psychiatric disorders:**
  - Bipolar disorders (More effective in acute mania)
  - Patients with poor response to lithium
  - Mixed affective disorder
  - Co-morbid substance use disorders
- **Neurological disorders:**
  - Seizure disorders (as an anticonvulsant)
  - Organic mania with seizure disorder
  - Patients with history of head injury
  - EEG abnormality
  - Migraine
  - Trigeminal neuralgia and neuropathic pain.

Side Effects

- Sedation, nausea, tremor, weight gain, hair loss, menstrual disturbance, thrombocytopenia, polycystic ovarian disease.
- Hepatic toxicity.
- Acute hemorrhagic pancreatitis.

Carbamazepine

Indications

- Psychiatric disorders (as mood stabilizer in bipolar disorder)
- Neurological disorder (seizures, pain syndromes/neuralgia).

Contraindications

Cardiac, renal and hepatic problems, bone marrow depression.

Side Effects

Some serious side effects are bone marrow depression that leads to aplastic anemia, agranulocytosis and cardiovascular collapse.

Diplopia, drowsiness, nausea, vomiting, ataxia, skin rashes, photosensitivity, cholestatic jaundice, leucopenia, thrombocytopenic purpura are other side effects.

ANTIANXIETY DRUGS (MINOR TRANQUILIZERS)

Anxiety is an important early symptom in many mental disorders. Drugs used to treat anxiety are called antianxiety agents (Anxiolytics). It is used to relieve moderate or severe anxiety in many physical disorders and emotional disorders like mild depression.

Indications

- To control withdrawal symptoms in alcoholism.
- To relieve anxiety associated with environmental stress.
- To control convulsions.
- To induce skeletal muscle relaxation.
- To enhance sleep and relaxation before investigations/surgery.

Mode of Action

These drugs enhance the action of gamma-aminobutyric acid (GABA), which is an inhibitory neurotransmitter. This inhibits the cortical and limbic system of brain which is involved in emotional reactions and anxiety.

Contraindications

Special precaution is needed in patients with liver or renal dysfunctions and respiratory impairment.

Classification

- **Barbiturates:** This group is not recommended for anxiety disorders.
- **Non-barbiturate non-benzodiazepines:** This group of drugs are also not used as antianxiety medicines.
- **Benzodiazepines:** These are the widely used antianxiety drug and had replaced other antianxiety drugs. These drugs are classified as per their half-lives. The drugs that are used in this class are shown in Table 6.6.

Table 6.6: Classification of benzodiazepines

Class and name of drug	*Dose of drug (mg/day)*
• Very short acting drug	
– Midazolam	Not used on psychiatric treatment
– Triazolam	Used as hypnotic
• Short acting drugs	
– Alprazolam	0.5–6 mg
– Lorazepam	2–6 mg orally OR 2–4 mg IV
– Oxazepam	15–120 mg
• Long acting drugs	
– Chlordiazepoxide	15–100 mg orally OR 50–100 mg IM/IV
– Clonazepam	0.5–20 mg orally OR 2–5 mg IM/IV
– Diazepam	2–30 mg orally OR 2–20 mg IM/IV
– Flurazepam	15–60 mg
– Nitrazepam	5–20 mg

ANTIPARKINSONIAN DRUGS

In psychiatry, these drugs are used to prevent or treat parkinsonian features that can occur as an extra pyramidal side effect of antipsychotics. Antiparkinsonian drugs include (Table 6.7):

- Anticholinergics decrease/block the secretion and reduce akathisia and dystonia.
- Antihistamines also has similar action.
- Dopaminergic drugs are dopamine releasing agents from the neurons.

Contraindications

Patients with:

- Hypersensitivity
- Closed angle glaucoma
- Prostatic hypertrophy
- Urinary or intestinal obstruction
- Tachycardia and cardiac problems.

Special precaution to be taken in patients with myasthenia gravis, and respiratory impairment.

Table 6.7: Drugs used as antiparkinsonian agents

Name of drug	*Dose (mg/day)*
• Anticholinergic drugs	
– Benztropine (cogentin)	0.5–60
– Biperiden HCL (akinetone)	2.0–8.0
– Trihexyphenidyl HCL (Pacitane, Parkin)	2.0–12.0
• Antihistamine	
– Diphen hydramine (benadryl)	75–100
• Dopaminergics	
– Bromocriptine	2.5–45
– Carbidopa/levodopa (sinemet)	10–100

Side Effects

- **Anticholinergic side effects** are—dry mouth, dry skin, blurred vision, photophobia, tachycardia, constipation, urinary retention, confusion.
- **Side effects of antihistamines** are—drowsiness, dizziness, anorexia, nausea, vomiting, orthostatic hypotension, weight gain, weakness.
- **Side effects of dopaminergic drugs** are—slurring of speech, poor concentration, dry mouth, mood changes, insomnia.

Nurse's Role

- Observation for side effects and desired effects like sedation, drowsiness, blurring of vision and tachycardia.
- Record vital signs in every four hours, and more frequently if needed
- Maintain intake-output chart. Assess for urinary retention
- Encourage adequate fluid intake
- Change the patient's position slowly and ambulate carefully
- Advise not to use hazardous machinery and driving.
- Advise to follow a planned routine
- Advise for regular eye check up if patient have blurring vision
- Educate the patient and the family about side effects, and nursing care aspects.

SOMATIC THERAPIES

Electroconvulsive Therapy (ECT)

ECT is an effective and specific treatment method for psychiatric disorders. The assumption that led to induction of seizure as a therapy are:

- Symptoms of schizophrenia often decreased after seizure
- Schizophrenia and epilepsy do not coexist in a person.

Initially seizure was induced in the treatment of psychosis with the help of camphor during 16th century. Then it was tried with the help of chemicals. In 1938, Italian psychiatrists Ugo Cerletti and Lucio Bini used ECT in the treatment of psychiatric disorders.

Definition

ECT is the artificial induction of generalized seizure by applying electrical current to brain with the help of electrodes that are placed either unilaterally or bilaterally.

Modified ECT

It is the induction of generalized seizure by applying electric current to brain with the help of electrodes, which is done under general anesthesia (GA). Use of GA and muscle relaxants made ECT more safe and acceptable.

Indications of ECT

The condition that indicates ECT as a first indication is major/severe depression. Main indications are:

- **Major depression with suicidal risk**
  - Severe depression with stupor and lack of food and fluid intake
  - Depression with psychotic features
  - Depression which is not responding to drug therapy
  - If drugs are contraindicated (some patients show severe side effects to drugs).
- **Catatonia**
  - Catatonic schizophrenia
  - Non-organic catatonia with stupor.
- **Severe psychosis**
  - Schizophrenia
  - Mania with psychotic features
  - Psychosis with suicide or homicide risk
  - Schizophrenia with severe depressive features.

Contraindications

Absolute contraindications for ECT is increased intracranial pressure which can occur secondary to several medical conditions like:

- Subarachnoid hemorrhage
- Subdural hemorrhage
- Brain tumors.

Relative contraindications are:

- History of recent myocardial infarction (within 3 months)
- Malignant hypertension
- Cerebrovascular accident (CVA)
- Pheochromocytoma
- Increased intraocular pressure/retinal detachment.

ECT Procedure

ECT is given by different techniques. It can be direct or modified.

- **Direct ECT:** Artificial induction of generalized seizure directly—without general anesthesia and muscle relaxant. Now it is not preferred.
- **Modified ECT:** It is the induction of generalized seizure along with the use of general anesthesia and muscle relaxant.

Based on the nature of electrode application, ECT can be bilateral/unilateral (Fig. 6.1 and 6.2).

Bilateral ECT

It is the commonest form of ECT, that is usually preferred and more effective than unilateral.

Electrodes are placed bilaterally—1½ inches above the midpoint of line drawn from the outer canthus of eye to the tragus of the ear.

Unilateral ECT

Electrodes are placed on one side of head, on the non-dominant side of brain (left side of head in a left handed person). Different positions are used for electrode placement.

Unilateral ECT have less side effects only. It is used in patients showing memory impairment after bilateral ECT.

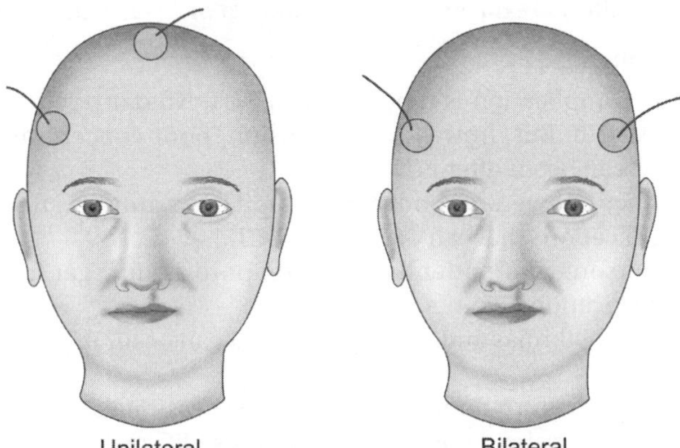

Fig. 6.1: Electrode placement in unilateral and bilateral ECT

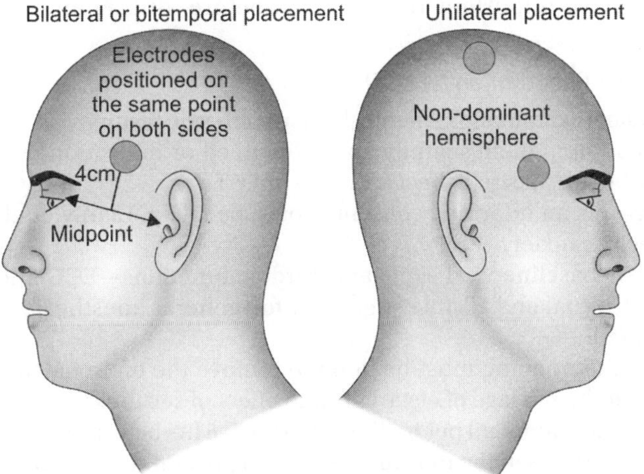

Fig. 6.2: Locating the site of electrodes in bilateral and unilateral ECT

Electrodes are placed after cleaning the site of electrode placement, an applying saline or electrode jelly, for better conduction of electricity. Dose of electrical current is 80–120 volts and duration is 0.1 to 1 second.

Effect of treatment is assessed by the occurrence of grand mal seizure and its duration as 30–60 seconds.

The principle of action of ECT is not clear, but it is assumed that there is some effect on catecholamine pathway between diencephalon and limbic system.

Number of ECT will vary with the nature of illness. Usually a total of 6–10 ECT in alternate days is given, maximum of 20–25 can be given.

Complications of ECT

No serious complication is reported with ECT. No damage to brain or its function also. But drowsiness, confusion, poor concentration and restlessness can occur after ECT.

Headache, fatigue and bodyache, palpitation and tongue bite are some complications that can occur after ECT.

Older persons and patients with osteoporosis may get fracture of bones or dislocation of joints.

Cardiac arrhythmias and respiratory arrest can occur in patients with heart disease.

ECT is a procedure done by a team of professionals—psychiatrist, anesthesiologist, trained nurse and sometimes EEG technician also.

Nurse's Role in ECT

Nurses have important role in ECT—before, during and after the procedure.

Before ECT (Preparation for ECT)

- Physical examination, medical and psychiatric history.
- Explain to patient's family about the need or indication of ECT, its side effects, desired effect and risks of ECT.
- After this an informed consent should be taken. Clarify doubts and alleviate anxiety.
- Assess baseline vital signs and cardiac functions—ECG and X-ray must be taken. All investigations for general anesthesia may be ordered.
- Hair shampooing must be done to remove the oil in hair, as it can hinder the passage of electricity and effect of seizure.
- Keep the patient nil per orally (NPO) for 4–6 hrs before ECT. Withhold the oral drugs in the morning of ECT (to prevent risk of vomiting and aspiration).

- Withhold the drugs with anticonvulsant action as it increases the seizure threshold and decrease the effect of seizure.
- Remove nail polish and lipstick, so that cyanosis can be observed clearly early.
- Remove all jewelry, dentures and other metallic objects and before shifting the patient to ECT room, to prevent electric shock.
- Remove artificial dentures to prevent its dislodgement and blockage of airway.
- Loose clothes must be given to ensure easy breathing.
- Ask the patient to empty bladder and bowel before ECT, to prevent incontinence during ECT which can occur due to use of muscle relaxant.
- Injection Atropine 0.6 mg IM is given 30 minutes before ECT, or given as IV on the table just before ECT to decrease the secretions and to prevent aspiration.
- Check the orders of anesthesiologist and complete all documentation before shifting patient to the ECT room.

Nurse's Role during ECT

- Place the patient on the ECT table in supine position.
- Be with the patient, so that he/she will feel secure without fear and anxiety.
- Administer anesthetic drug—thiopental sodium (3-5 mg/kg body weight) and muscle relaxant—succinylcholine (1 mg/kg body weight).
- Ventilatory support must begin from the time of administration of muscle relaxant as it paralyzes all the muscles including respiratory muscles.
- Keep a mouth gag between the rows of teeth, to prevent tongue bite.
- The site of electrode placement is cleaned or moistened with normal saline or electrode jelly, which helps in better conduction of electricity.
- Voltage, duration of electrical stimulus and seizure activity with its duration should be monitored (apply BP cuff to one of the lower extremities, just before the administration of muscle relaxant. This helps in monitoring the duration of seizure activity as the presence of jerks in that limb. Application of BP cuff helps to occlude the muscle relaxant, so that limb will show jerky movement during seizure).
- Support major joints—shoulder and arm and restraint thighs to prevent dislocation.

- During the procedure, monitor ECG and oxygen saturation. Sometimes EEG also may be recorded. Duration of seizure must be recorded. 100% oxygen is administered during the procedure.
- Record all the details—medications, voltage, duration of seizure, vital signs and ECG changes.

Post ECT Care

- Monitor vital signs—especially rate and depth of respiration and ECG.
- Keep the patient in side lying position and keep the airway clean. If needed suction must be done to clear the airway.
- Oxygen through mask to be continued for at least half an hour or till respiration and oxygen saturation becomes normal.
- Assess the level of consciousness and orientation. Sometimes the patient may be restless and disoriented. So keep him/her in a bed with side rails.
- Some patients may show confusion and/or impairment in memory. So reorient him/her to environment. There will be muscle pain all over the body and headache.
- Once the patient becomes fully conscious, can give oral sips of clear fluids and observe for chocking. Then give clear fluids.
- Careful ambulation is important to prevent falls and injury.
- Help the patient in activities of daily living.

Insulin Shock Therapy

It was introduced by Sakel in 1933 in treating schizophrenia. Large dose of insulin is injected to produce hypoglycemia in the patient and thus patient goes to coma after some time. IV injection of 25% glucose is given to get up patient within 10–20 minutes. This procedure needs constant observation. Now it is not used.

Psychosurgery

Lobotomy is the surgical procedure that severe the interconnecting fibers between the parts of brain and thus to decrease or stimulate brain tissue. This will help in modifying thought, mood and behavior. It was preferred when all other measures are not effective. Leucotomy was the first psychosurgery and was done by Egas Moniz and Almenda Lima in 1936. In 1937, prefrontal lobotomy was made. Due to public criticism it is not used now.

Light Therapy

It is the use of artificial light (2500 lux for 1–2 hrs daily) in the treatment of seasonal affective disorder. Individual is asked to directly look at the light in every few minutes. Therapeutic effect is mediated by the eyes.

- **Indications:** Seasonal affective disorder, bulimia nervosa.
- **Contraindications:** Glaucoma, cataract, use of drug that cause photosensitivity.
- **Adverse effects:** Headache, eye irritation.

Transcranial Magnetic Stimulation

Activity of brain is influenced by producing a magnetic field over the brain. It acts by increasing the release of neurotransmitters and by down regulation of beta adrenergic receptors and resolves the depressive features.

Adverse effects are seizure in persons without previous history of it. Transient hearing loss and headache are some other side effects. Patients with pacemaker or other metal implants, cardiac problems and increased intracranial pressure need special precautions.

PSYCHOSOCIAL THERAPY

Introduction

The treatment approaches used for psychiatric patients are psychopharmacology, psychosocial therapies and somatic therapy. Psychosocial therapies are mainly employed for patients with behavioral problems and for problems which arise out of psychosocial factors.

PSYCHOTHERAPY

Definition

Psychotherapy is defined as a treatment by psychological means of problems of emotional nature in which the therapist establishes a professional relationship with the patient to:

- Remove or modify the existing symptoms
- Mediate disturbed patterns of behavior
- Promote positive personality growth and development (Wolberg).

Psychotherapy is a method of treatment based on the development of therapeutic relationship between the client and therapist for the purpose of exploring and modifying the client's behavior in a satisfying direction (Lego S).

Goals of Psychotherapy

- Modify the maladaptive behavior
- Develop self-awareness and improve self-esteem
- Helps in the resolution of inner conflicts
- Fosters communication and interpersonal skills.

Types of Psychotherapy

Types of psychotherapy are shown in Flowchart 6.1.

Flowchart 6.1: Types of psychotherapy

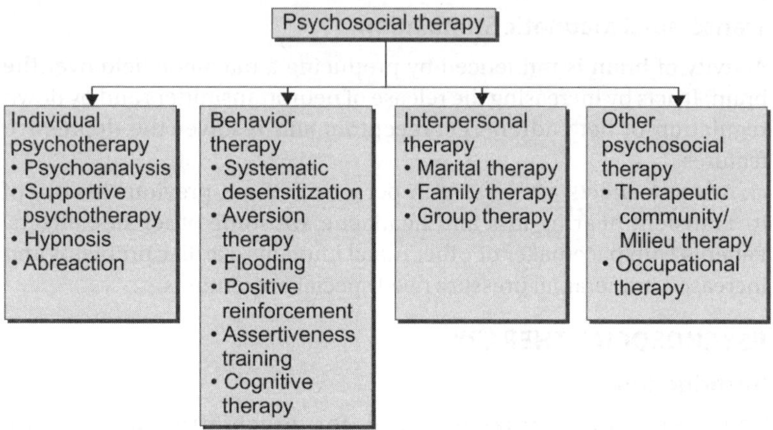

Individual Psychotherapy

This type of psychotherapy is conducted on one-to-one basis.

Psychoanalysis

This therapy was developed by Sigmund Freud. Psychoanalysis as a therapy focuses on the influence of repressed feelings and internal conflicts on the behavior of an individual. It is a technique in which the patient is allowed to ventilate whatever is coming to his mind. The client will be made to lie on a soft coach in a relaxed manner. The distractions are minimized and the patient will be allowed to communicate. The role of the therapist is an active listener and no advice is given to the patient. Techniques used in psychoanalysis are free association, working through the repressed feelings and its interpretation.

Free association is a technique in which person reveals emotions or impulses whatever comes to his/her mind regardless of whether they are socially unacceptable.

Aims of Psychoanalysis

- To relieve anxiety
- To identify behavioral deviation
- To preserve mental health

Supportive Psychotherapy

It is a type of psychotherapy in which support is offered to the patient as a friend, philosopher or guide. In this the therapist helps the patient to relieve his emotional distress.

Indications

- Acute life crisis
- Schizophrenia
- Depression
- Acute stress reaction
- Mental retardation
- Childhood psychiatric disorder.

Purpose of Supportive Psychotherapy

- It helps to strengthens ego
- It provides support for a person when in distress
- Helps to improve the confidence
- Helps to deal with the situation in an effective manner.

Techniques of Supportive Psychotherapy

- **Ventilation:** It is technique in which patient is allowed to express feelings and emotions freely. This will make the person much relaxed as he was able to talk about his feelings.
- **Environmental manipulation:** Involves changing the environment so as to promote the mental health of the person. Example: A patient who was not able to sleep due to restlessness of another patient, the restless patient may be shifted to another room.
- **Re-education:** Educating the family members about the role in the treatment of mentally ill.
- **Reassurance:** Emotional support is given to individuals experiencing distress.
- **Persuasion:** This involves compelling the client to change or modify his behavior.
- **Guidance:** It involves offering suggestions to the patient to deal with the difficult situation.

Hypnosis

It is superficial or deep sleep-like state (trance) produced by giving suggestions and making him concentrate on a single object. During hypnosis, the person will be suggestible and he can be made to recall repressed events and thus helps to gain relief from anxiety.

Abreaction

Refers to therapeutic technique in which patient talks about repressed emotions. Expression of unconscious material will help to reduce the underlying fear or anxiety.

Behavioral Therapy

It is a type of psychotherapy based on theories of learning, aims at changing the maladaptive behavior in an adaptive behavior.

Aims of Behavioral Therapy

- To change the maladaptive into adaptive one
- Correction of abnormal psychodynamics
- Helpful in conditions which are refractory to other forms of therapy.

Indications of Behavioral Therapy

- Anxiety disorders
- Phobia
- Post-traumatic stress disorder
- Obsessive-compulsive disorder
- Bipolar mood disorder
- Depression
- Schizophrenia
- Somatoform disorder
- Eating disorder
- Dissociative disorder
- Psychosomatic disorder
- Sexual disorder
- Substance abuse
- Childhood disorder
- Dementia.

Types of Behavioral Therapy

- Systematic desensitization
- Flooding
- Aversion therapy
- Operant conditioning to increase the behavior
- Operant conditioning to decrease the behavior
- Assertiveness training
- Cognitive therapy.

Systematic Desensitization

This therapy was developed by J Wolpe. The goal of the therapy is to reduce fear of a person by exposing him to the feared object in a graded manner.

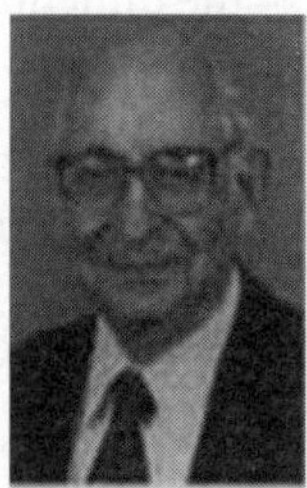

Joseph Wolpe

Indications
- Phobia
- Obsessive-compulsive disorder
- Anxiety.

Steps in systematic desensitization: The steps involved in systematic desensitization are:
- **Relaxation training:** The patient is trained to relax by deep breathing, meditation or progressive muscle relaxation.
- **Hierarchy construction:** Asking the patient to construct a hierarchy of the situation producing anxiety.
- **Desensitization proper:** The patient is exposed to the stimulus either in imagery or in reality. The lowest item in the hierarchy is confronted either in imagery or in reality. The patient is instructed to signal whenever anxiety occurs. With each signal the patient is instructed to relax, after few trials the patient is able to control his anxiety. The therapy is continued till the maximum anxiety is attained and the stimulus can be faced with no anxiety (Fig. 6.3).

Flooding

It is a type of behavioral therapy in which patient is exposed to phobic situation in a non-graded manner from which escape is impossible. By prolonged exposure with phobic stimulus, anxiety gradually decreased with therapist's guidance and encouragement.

Indications: Phobia, Anxiety, and obsessive-compulsive disorder.

Aversion Therapy

In this pleasant stimulus (alcohol) is paired with an unpleasant response, so that even in the absence of unpleasant response, the pleasant stimulus becomes unpleasant by association.

Indications
- Alcoholism
- Sexual disorders
- Homosexuality
- Transvestism.

Operant Conditioning to Increase the Behavior
- **Positive reinforcement:** The desirable behavior is reinforced by reward either symbolic or material (Fig. 6.4).
- **Negative reinforcement:** On the performance of a desirable behavior punishment can be avoided.
- **Modeling:** Here the person is instructed to copy or model the behavior of the therapist.

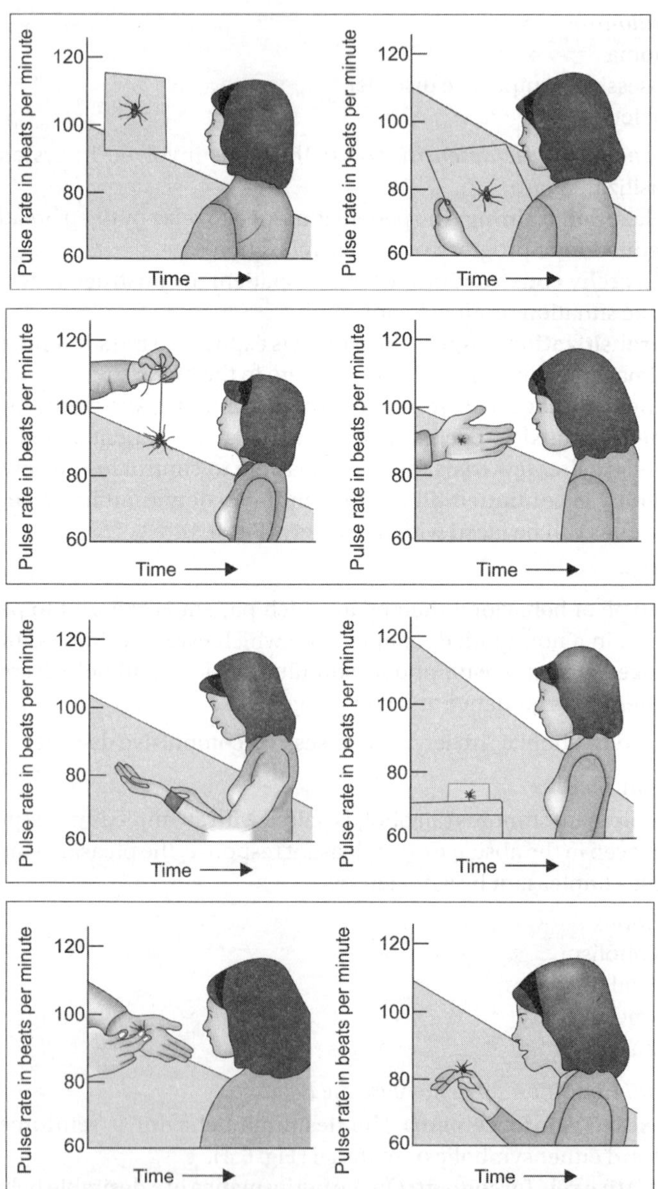

Fig. 6.3: Graded exposure for a client who has phobia towards spider

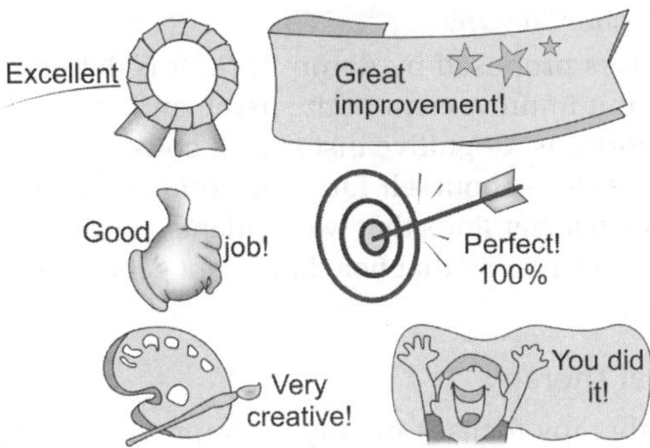

Fig. 6.4: Types of positive reinforcement

Operant Conditioning to Decrease the Behavior

- **Time out:** Here the child is withdrawn for some time, e.g. the child is not allowed to go out for play if he fails to complete the task (Fig. 6.5).
- **Punishment:** Whenever an undesired behavior occurs punishment is given.
- **Token economy:** It is a type of behavioral therapy in which reinforcement is mainly by token to be exchanged for privileges (Fig. 6.6).

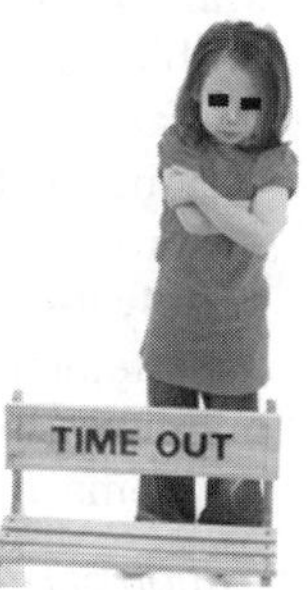

Fig. 6.5: Time out

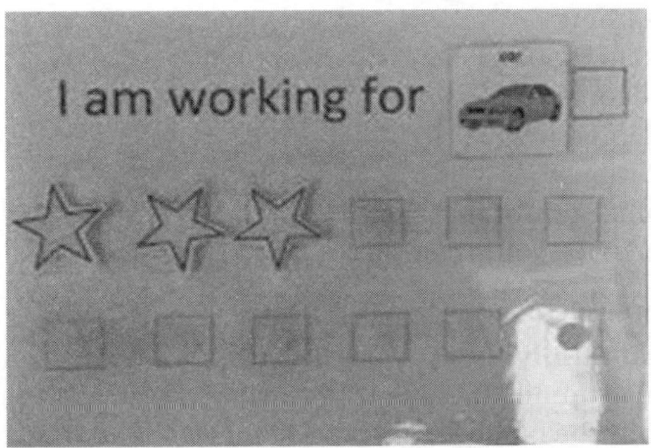

Fig. 6.6: Token economy

Assertiveness Training

It is a training given to the patient or person to encourage direct but socially acceptable thoughts and feelings by people who are shy. It was first described by Salter and develops by Wolpe. The indications include depression and social phobia.

Cognitive Behavior Therapy

This therapy was proposed by Aaron Beck. It is defined as a therapy which brings out improvement in the psychiatric illness by correcting cognitive distortions. Cognitive distortions consist of thoughts which involve negative views about self, future or world. Example for a cognitive distortion—the teacher finds that two students are getting bored in the class and she may assume that her class is not good. Used as treatment for depression.

Interpersonal Therapy

This type of therapy focuses mainly on improving the interpersonal relationship. This includes:

- **Marital therapy/couple therapy:** Whenever there is relationship problems couple therapy is considered. The couple together visit the family therapist and the therapist will observe their interaction, communication, hopes and expectations and suggest ways to solve the problems.
- **Family therapy:** It is a type of psychotherapy that focuses on altering the interactions between couples within a nuclear family or between members in an extended family with the goal of alleviating the problems of the individual family members in the family subsystem.

Indication of Family Therapy

- Schizophrenia
- Mood disorders
- Relationship problems
- Reactive depression
- Anxiety depression
- Substance abuse
- Psychosomatic disorder
- Childhood psychiatric disorder.

Types of Family Therapy

- **Individual family therapy:** In this each individual members will have a single family therapist. They will work out on specific issues, occasionally the family members will meet alone with therapist.
- **Single family therapy:** Here the family therapist will observe the family interactions and help the family members to clearly define the problems and suggest ways to overcome the problem. The suggested activities will be carried out and then modified if needed.
- **Multiple family group therapy:** In this 4–5 families meet weekly to discuss about the common problems.

- **Psychoeducation:** Information regarding the psychiatric diagnosis, treatment and the role of family in the various therapies is given.

Nurse's Role in Family Therapy

The nurse has to assess the family structure, past medical and mental illness, communication and family interactions. Nurses can provide counseling, motivate the family to improve listening skills, involve the family members in the provision of care and arrange for community resources.

Group Therapy

Definition

Group psychotherapy or group therapy is a form of psychotherapy in which one or more therapists treat a small group of clients together as a group.

Group therapy is a form of psychotherapy that involves sessions guided by a therapist and attended by persons who face similar problems.

Types of Group Therapy

- **Therapeutic group therapy:** Refers to therapy in which a group of patients work together to promote their mental health under the supervision of therapist, e.g. group of postnatal mothers, patients with diabetes or cancer.
- **Adjunctive group therapy:** Addresses the special interests of a group, e.g. art therapy is given for self-expression.
- **Encounter group or T group:** A person gains awareness regarding his own feelings and behavior towards others. It is not necessary that the group members are patients.
- **Homogenous group and heterogeneous group:** Homogenous group is composed of patients of same age, sex and disease. In heterogeneous group, members differ in all these characteristics.
- **Open groups and closed groups:** Open groups permit the group member to enter or leave the group at any time. Closed groups have a specified number of people and have fixed schedule.
- **Self-help groups:** These groups are organized by patients who have recovered from mental illness or by relatives of the affected person. The group members often share their experience of adjusting with the problems and thus the other members can practice similar ways. Examples include alcoholic anonymous, parents of autistic children.

Goals of Group Therapy

- Improves communication
- Develops insight

- Promotes personal growth
- Encourages creative expression.

Indications of Group Therapy

- Depression
- Substance abuse
- Domestic violence
- Eating disorders.

Group Therapy Process

Group therapy involves certain steps which include:

- **Selecting the group members and leader:** The therapist has to determine the criteria for the inclusion of the group members. The optimum size should be 8–10. It is also desired that the group members share common problems or interests.
- **Conducting group therapy sessions:** The therapist has to decide the venue and time of meeting. The purpose of the group session, frequency and the responsibilities of each member have to be clearly specified. It is important that confidentiality is maintained. Members have to be instructed to be punctual and to have free communication.

Role of Group Leader or Nurse in Group Therapy

- Decision to establish a group
- Provide information
- Encourages ventilation of feelings
- Improves communication and socialization skills
- Set limits to patient's behavior
- Act as a role model
- Suggest ways to overcome a problem.

Milieu Therapy

Definition

The total resources of the staff, the resident, and their relatives and the institution is pooled for the purpose of treatment (Maxwell Jones).

A therapy in which the client's social environment has to be changed, to provide a therapeutic experience for the patient by involving him as an active participant in their own care and to deal with the daily problems of his community.

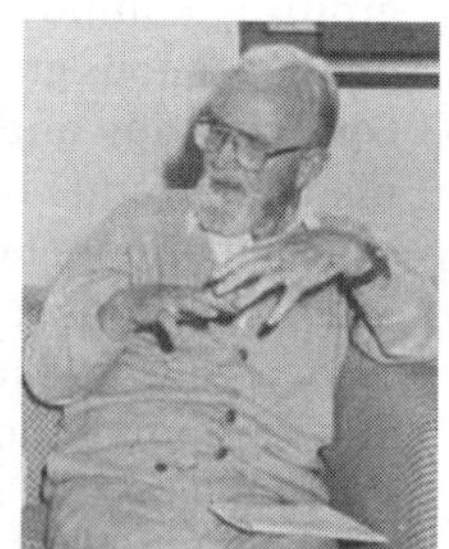

Maxwell Jones

Goals of Milieu Therapy

- Changes maladaptive behavior into adaptive behavior.
- Provides a favorable environment.

- Minimizes prolongation of hospital stay.
- Promotes early recovery.
- Encourages the client to participate activities of daily living.
- Improves self-esteem.
- Promotes self-confidence.
- Promotes social interaction.

Indications

- Alcohol use disorder
- Depression
- Neurosis
- Somatoform disorder.

Features

- Informal atmosphere—clients can have communication which is open and free.
- Mutual therapeutic environment.
- Shared decision making—clients as well as the staff can make decisions.
- Residents play an active role—management of the environment is mainly by the clients.
- Regular community meetings—importance is given to interaction of the staff as well as the clients.
- Feedback—residents are allowed to give feedback regarding each intervention.
- Limit setting—It is important that the nurse has to set limits.
- Minimize environmental stressors.

Principles

- Democratization—the therapy is comprised of the clients carried out by them for their welfare.
- Permissiveness—it gives freedom for the clients in decision making.
- Reality confrontation—clients often have to face and cope with their problems.
- Group activity—milieu therapy is focused on group work.
- Decision making—improves the self-esteem of the client.

Team Members

- Psychiatrist
- Clinical psychologist
- Psychiatric clinical nurse specialist
- Psychiatric social worker
- Occupational therapist

- Recreational therapist
- Music therapist
- Art therapist
- Psychodramatist
- Chaplain.

Advantages

- Develops good interpersonal relationship
- Improves self-confidence
- Promotes socialization skills
- Encourages collective thinking.

Disadvantages

- Lack of responsibility
- Role confusion.

Role of Nurse in Milieu Therapy

Maxwell Jones, the proponent of milieu therapy has identified 3 roles for the nurse (Tripartite role):

1. **Authoritarian Role:** Here the nurse has to set limits to the client's behavior and controls the group.
2. **Social Role:** The nurse promotes the communication and interpersonal relationships
3. **Therapeutic Role:** Nurse involves actively in the treatment approaches by administering medicines, involving in other therapies and also by maintaining relationship.

Occupational Therapy

Definition

Occupational therapy refers to the use of goal-oriented, purposeful activity in the assessment and treatment of individuals with psychological, physical or developmental disabilities.

World federation of occupational therapists defined occupational therapy as a profession concerned with promoting health and well-being through occupation.

Goals of Occupational Therapy

- Identify the interests and skills of the client.
- Remove behaviors that hinder with occupational performance.
- Improve the job performance.
- Assist the client to develop skills.

- Encourage independence in daily activities.
- Improve self-esteem.
- Enhances physical coordination.

Categories of Occupational Therapy

- Activity therapy
- Vocational training.

Activities in Occupational Therapy

- Relaxation techniques
- Yoga
- Walking, jogging
- Dance
- Quiz
- Creative writing
- Art and poetry.

Vocational Training

Once the client regains physical strengths and emotional state, he will be given training in the following jobs:

- Basket making
- Candle making
- Craft work
- Sewing
- Jewelry making
- Gardening.

Steps Involved in Occupational Therapy

- Evaluate the abilities, strengths and limitations of the client.
- Set goals
- Develop the treatment plan
- Implement the treatment plan
- Evaluate the plan
- Set future goals based on evaluation.

Settings for Occupational Therapy Units

- Psychiatric hospital
- Rehabilitation center
- Day care centers
- Industrial health unit
- Special home for children
- Community mental health center.

CONCLUSION

Most people experience different kinds of problems in their lives which may sometimes affect their mental health. Psychosocial therapies are effective in these situations as well as with mentally ill. Awareness regarding psychosocial therapies is needed for the nurse in promoting mental health and prevention of mental illness.

Psychotropic drugs and ECT have important role in the management of psychiatric disorders. Nurses are the most responsible persons in these therapies, as they are in the wards throughout day and night and observes the patients for their distress/side effects and desired effects also. Along with this nurses can educate the relatives and the patient regarding the need of regular treatment and follow up. For this nurses must have good knowledge about action, indications, contraindications, side effects and its management and specific care with each group of drugs.

BIBLIOGRAPHY

1. Ahuja N. A Short Textbook of Psychiatry (Seventh edition). New Delhi: Jaypee Brothers Medical Publishers (P) Ltd, 2011.
2. Kapoor B. Textbook of Psychiatric Nursing. Delhi: Kumar Publishing House, 2014.
3. Manisha Gupta. A Textbook of Therapeutic Modalities in Psychiatric Nursing. Jaypee Brothers Medical Publishers (P) Ltd, 2015.
4. Sadock BJ, Sadock VA, Ruiz P. Kaplan and Sadock's Synopsis of Psychiatry: Behavioral Sciences/Clinical Psychiatry (Ninth edition). Philadelphia: Wolters Kluwer, 2009.
5. Sreevani R. Psychology for Nurses (Second edition). New Delhi: Jaypee Brothers Medical Publishers (P) Ltd, 2013.
6. Stuart GW, Laraia MT. Principles and Practice of Psychiatric Nursing. St Louis: Mosby, 2001.
7. Townsend CM. Psychiatric Mental Health Nursing: Concepts of Care in Evidence-based Practice (7th edition). Philadelphia: FA Davis Company, 2012.
8. Vyas JN, Ghimire RS. Textbook of Postgraduate Psychiatry (Third edition). New Delhi: Jaypee Brothers Medical Publishers (P) Ltd, 2016.

CHAPTER 7

Organic Mental Disorders

INTRODUCTION

Etiology of mental disorders are widely accepted as Biopsychosocial factors. Biological factors include organic causes, which are demonstrable in investigations. The type of mental disorders due to organic causes are considered as organic mental disorders.

As per DSM V this group is classified as neurocognitive disorders (NCD) and include delirium, mild and major neurocognitive disorders.

DEFINITION

Organic mental disorders are psychological or behavioral disturbances due to deficit in cognition, that is associated with brain dysfunctions that are demonstrable in investigations.

Some characteristic features that may indicate organicity are:

- Old age person with first episode of acute onset.
- History of psychoactive substance abuse.
- Coexisting illness, especially neurological disorder.
- History of epilepsy, alteration of consciousness, sensory or motor problems.
- History of head injury.
- Soft neurological signs with cognitive impairment.
- Non-auditory hallucinations (usually, visual, tactile, olfactory or gustatory).

CLASSIFICATION–ICD 10

F00-F09 Organic including Symptomatic Mental Disorders

- F00: Dementia in Alzheimers disease
- F01: Vascular dementia
- F04: Organic amnestic syndrome
- F05: Delirium
- F06: Other mental disorders due to brain damage and dysfunction and physical disease.

- F07: Personality and behavioral disorders due to brain diseases, damage and dysfunction.

Most commonly seen subcategories of organic mental disorders are:

- Delirium.
- Dementia.
- Organic amnestic syndrome.

DELIRIUM

Delirium is the most common organic mental disorder and occurrence is high in patients in intensive care units. Disturbance in attention and change in cognition develop rapidly in a short period.

Definition

It is a mental state of clouding of consciousness, with disturbance in cognition and manifested as confusion, excitement/restlessness, disorientation, illusion and hallucination.

Epidemiology

The prevalence of delirium in community is comparatively low (1–2%) as compared to hospitalized patients (10–31%). In intensive care units (ICU), prevalence is 80% and in postoperative ICU, 10–70%.

In India prevalence of delirium is 3–27% in hospitalized patients of more than 65 years.

Clinical Features

Delirium usually occurs suddenly after a neurologic problem like head injury or seizure. It may occur after several days or hours of restlessness, insomnia or somnolence and difficulty in thinking.

Clinical features are:

- Acute onset of clouding of consciousness
- Restlessness and extreme distractibility
- Disorganized thinking, observable as irrelevant, pressured, and incoherent speech with sudden topic change.
- Inability to do goal directed activity due to poor attention span.
- Disorientation to time and place.
- Impairment in immediate and recent memory.
- Disturbance in perception (Illusion and Hallucination—usually of non-auditory).
- Disturbance in sleep wake cycle as diurnal variation with worsening of symptoms in night.

- Increased psychomotor activity—as restlessness, purposeless movement, or tremor. Screaming, muttering, activities as harming self or others.
- Other motor symptoms that are specific to delirium are:
  - *Carphologia or Floccilation* (picking movements at sheets and clothes).
  - *Asterixis or Flapping tremor.*
- Emotional instability/labile affect expressed as fear, anxiety, anger or irritability.
- Autonomic disturbances as tachycardia, increased blood pressure, sweating and dilated pupil.
- Speech problems are slurring, dysarthria and incoherence.

Delirium is usually reversible or transient with a duration of 1 week, or may extend up to 1 month. Rarely it may persist as a permanent cognitive disorder.

Etiology

Postoperative patients and people with neuro problems are more prone to develop delirium. Etiological factors include predisposing factors and some specific etiologic factors.

Predisposing factors are:

- Cerebral lesions as brain abscess or stroke.
- Seizures.
- Extremes of age—as being very old or young.
- Febrile illness.
- Metabolic disorders and other chronic medical illness (hepatic or renal).
- Head injury.
- Migraine headache.
- Treatment with psychotropic drugs.

Etiology of Delirium

Etiology can be single factor as in case of alcohol withdrawal or can be described under the following headings:

- **Intracranial causes:** Epilepsy, intracranial infections like meningitis, encephalitis, etc.
- **Metabolic causes:** Hypoxia, hypoglycemia, uremic encephalopathy, hepatic encephalopathy, electrolyte imbalance, etc.
- **Intoxication:** Intoxication with substances like alcohol, cannabis, stimulants, and psychotropic drugs.
- **Withdrawal of substances:** Withdrawal from psychoactive substances like alcohol, opioids, etc.

- **Drug induced delirium:** Drugs like anticholinergics, antihypertensives, corticosteroids, anesthetics, antineoplastic drugs, antiparkinsonian drugs, etc. can cause delirium.
- **Systemic infections** like septicemia pneumonia, etc.
- **Other causes** include sleep deprivation and endocrine causes as hypo or hypersecretion from thyroid, parathyroid and adrenal glands.

Diagnosis

Diagnosis of delirium is usually based on clinical features. But lab tests are essential in identifying the etiology (e.g. increased blood urea in uremic encephalopathy).

Important diagnostic features include:

- Impairment in level of consciousness and attention which may vary from simple clouding of consciousness to coma.
- Global disturbance in cognition.
- Disturbance in psychomotor activities.
- Sleep wake cycle disturbance.

Lab tests include serum creatinine to rule out renal disease, liver function tests, thyroid function tests, serum electrolytes, investigation to assess intoxication also will be helpful. Radiological tests also may be needed.

Management

A detailed history collection will help in identifying the etiology. All essential blood investigations must be done to rule out the definite etiology or predisposing factor because the medical and nursing management must be based on specific etiology. (Urinalysis, blood investigations and radio diagnostic studies must be done.)

Once the etiology is identified, the underlying pathology can be corrected.

For example, oxygen is administered in case of hypoxia and correction of electrolyte in case of electrolyte imbalance, correction of hypoglycemia.

Small doses of lorazepam are the usual drug of choice. Antipsychotics to manage agitated patients with hallucination.

Effective management of underlying medical conditions can reverse delirium within 1–2 weeks or within 1 month.

Prognosis: Prognosis of delirium is good, especially if the basic etiology is identified and treated promptly. Delirium is reversible within a period of 1–2 weeks.

Nursing Considerations

Observation

- Vigilant observation and assessment from the nurse's part is important. Along with assessment, do the history collection also.
- Physical examination with more focus on neurological assessment.
- Closely observe for any injury or hematoma
- Observe for clinical features and vital signs. If possible can continuous monitoring of ECG and oxygen saturation. Assist with all necessary investigations.

Safety Precautions

- Prevent accidents and falls by ensuring safety. Keep the patient in a bed with side rails, if needed padded side rails.
- Provide safe environment, by removing all hazardous objects like sharp instruments and chemicals.
- Provide low stimuli environment, by providing a calm and quiet area in the ward. Preferably bed nearer to nurse's station or in ICU.
- Be calm and patient in your approach. Avoid arguments and shouting, though patient is restless/irritable.
- Be with the patient or ensure that somebody is with the patient, to protect patient and others.
- Keep the room or environment minimally furnished and well-lighted. Keep only essential things in room.

Reassurance

Reassure the patient by frequent orientation and relatives by helping them in reducing anxiety and fear with adequate explanation.

Ensure Basic Needs and Physical Well-being

- Assess patient's hygiene, nutrition and hydration along with physical examination.
- Assist in meeting hygienic needs if individual is able to follow instructions; otherwise provide total care, as in care of an unconscious patient—including care of skin and mouth, and meeting elimination needs in bed.
- Monitor vital signs, intake output and investigations—any abnormality should be immediately reported.

Ensure Adequate Rest and Sleep

Provide low stimuli environment with good ventilation and dim light. Comfortable bed with side rails, if needed comfort measures also. Avoid coffee and tea in late evening or before bedtime.

Improving Cognitive Functions

- Nursing care must focus on improving the cognitive abilities. Frequently assess orientation and reorient him or her to surroundings—time, date, day, month, place, person.
- Introduce the relatives nearby and the staff on duty.
- As far as possible, permit patient's belongings in the hospital.
- Keep a big clock and calendar in the room or nearby.

DEMENTIA

Dementia was known as chronic brain syndrome due to its slow progression, and presence of a group of symptoms. Most of the types of dementia are irreversible. Unlike delirium here patient is conscious or alert.

Definition

Dementia is a chronic, progressive organic mental disorder with global impairment in cognitive and executive functions, in the presence of consciousness and reflected as impairment in memory, intellectual ability and personality deterioration. As disease progresses, it will affect all activities of daily living.

DSM-V classification mentioned it as neurocognitive disorder (NCD)—mild or major based on the severity of symptoms.

Neurocognitive disorders are broadly classified as primary and secondary.

- Primary are those in which NCD will be the main sign of disorder.
- Secondary there will be some underlying disease like endocrine disorders, AIDS (Acquired Immunodeficiency Syndrome), head injury.

Epidemiology

In 2010, the global prevalence of dementia was 35.6 million. In India, prevalence is 3.7 million. Among the states of India, Thiruvananthapuram of Kerala and Tirupur of Tamil Nadu had the highest rates.

Clinical Features

- Recent memory is affected first. Individuals unable to learn new things.
- Usually slowly progressing and irreversible features (can be reversed in early stage if primary etiology is treated promptly).
- Impairment in intelligence, judgment, abstract thinking and impulse control. But consciousness is not affected.
- Thought disorder like delusions—mainly persecutory delusion.

- Emotional lability (rapidly fluctuating emotional expressions as irritability, anxiety or aggression).
- Catastrophic reactions (when something is assigned beyond intellectual capacity of client, he/she will feel raged and confused).
- Disorientation to time first and then to place and person towards later stages.
- Sleep wake pattern will be changed. 'sun downing' occurs towards later stages (symptoms seems to worsen during late afternoon and evening).
- Patient may be dysphoric/depressed, agitating and hallucinating as the stage advances.
- Neurological signs may or may not be there, based on the underlying etiology.
- Communication becomes difficult and may progress to aphasia.
- Apraxia (inability to carry out motor activities in the absence of motor dysfunctions) and agnosia (loss of comprehension of sensations, in the presence of intact sensory functions) are common as the course advances.

Etiology and Types of Dementia

There is no definite etiology in some cases of dementia as it occurs with ageing. Many conditions can lead to development of dementia and based on etiology, dementia can be classified also (Table 7.1).

Table 7.1: Types of dementia, based on etiology

Causes of dementia	*Types of dementia*
1. Parenchymatous brain disease	1. Primary degenerative dementia
2. Vascular changes leading to multiinfarct areas in brain	2. Vascular dementia
3. Head injury	3. Traumatic dementia
4. Substance intoxication/drug/heavy metal intoxication	4. Toxic dementia
5. Dementia due to AIDS	5. AIDS dementia complex.
6. Chronic hepatic and renal diseases leading to uremic encephalopathy and dementia	6. Metabolic dementia
7. Deficiency of vitamins	7. Deficiency dementia
8. Intracranial space occupying lesions	8. Neoplastic dementia

Types of Dementia

- **Dementia due to parenchymatous brain disease (primary degenerative dementia)**
  - *Dementia of alzheimer's type:* This is the most common type of dementia. Definite etiology is not known.

CT and MRI of brain shows degenerative changes as atrophy, widening of central sulci and dilated ventricles.

In microscopic study, there is neurofibrillary tangles and senile plaques in brain, and it rapidly increases. The tangles interfere the neuronal transport system and causes destruction or death of neurons. This neuronal loss lead to loss of memory, personality changes and other features.

Also there is a marked reduction in production of neurotransmitter—acetylcholine in brain and thus decreased neurotransmission in the cortex and hippocampus, causes cognitive impairment.

- **Dementia due to Parkinson's disease:** Loss of neurons in substantia nigra and decreased dopamine activity will lead to parkinsonian features and many of these patients have dementia also.
- **Dementia due to Pick's disease:** This is due to atrophy in the frontal and temporal lobes of the brain. Symptoms are similar to that of alzheimer's type.
- **Dementia due to Creutzfeldt-Jakob disease:** This is caused by a transmissible agent known as a 'slow virus.' Course of illness is extremely rapid, with progressive deterioration.
- **Dementia due to Huntington's disease:** Here damage occurs in the basal ganglia and areas of cerebral cortex. The average duration of the disease is based on age at onset.
- **Lewy body dementia:** Clinical feature are same as that of alzheimer's disease, but progress more rapidly. Early appearance of visual hallucinations and parkinsonian features are typical.

• **Vascular dementia (multi-infarct dementia):** This is the second commonest type and more common in men and with abrupt onset. Occurs due to cerebrovascular problems that interrupts the blood flow to specific area of brain and results in damage to the neurons in that area. Problems usually begin as muscular weakness and change in gait and memory problems usually occur later. Difficulty in speech also is there.

• **Dementia due to head injury:** Amnesia is the most common symptom along with confusion and problems in speech, vision and personality. These symptoms sometimes become permanent.

• **Substance/drug induced dementia:** Dementia caused by substance reactions and its overuse. Cognitive impairment persists even after the usual period of intoxication and sudden withdrawal of psychoactive substance or heavy metal poisoning (lead or mercury) or drug poisoning.

- **Dementia due to HIV infection (AIDS dementia complex):** Dementia is caused by either HIV type 1 itself or due to immune system dysfunction from HIV infection.
  Dementia can develop secondary to chronic infections like neurosyphilis, viral encephalitis, meningitis, etc.
- **Dementia due to metabolic disorders:** Chronic hepatic and renal diseases can cause uremic encephalopathy and may lead to dementia.
- **Dementia due to nutritional deficiency:** As the result of deficiency diseases like pernicious anemia, pellagra and due to deficiency of thiamin and folic acid deficiency.
- **Dementia due to neoplasms:** Dementia may occur with intracranial space occupying lesions.
- **Dementia due to other medical condition:** Endocrine disorders especially hypothyroidism, other thyroid, parathyroid, adrenal and pituitary dysfunctions, epilepsy, systemic lupus erythematosus (SLE), multiple sclerosis can lead to dementia.

Diagnosis

Investigations should be to rule out the specific causes. Lab investigations include—blood count, blood sugar, serum electrolytes, renal function tests, thyroid function test, serological tests, lumbar puncture and cerebrospinal fluid study, arterial blood analysis.

Other investigations are chest X-ray, EEG, skull X-ray, CT scan and MRI scan of brain and urinalysis.

Steps in diagnosis are:

- **Physical assessment**
- **Neuropsychological tests (mini mental status examination (MMSE)**
- **Lab Investigations:** Blood count, blood sugar, serum electrolytes, renal function tests, liver function tests, thyroid function test, serological tests, lumbar puncture, arterial blood analysis and urinalysis.
  Lumbar puncture to rule out infection of central nervous system.
- **Electroencephalogram (EEG)**
- **Radio diagnostic studies:** X-ray skull, CT scan, MRI scan of brain, PET to assess metabolic activity of brain.

Treatment

Specific drugs of choice in mild to moderate cases of dementia are cholinesterase inhibitors which in turn increases the acetylcholine.

Example: Tacrine hydrochloride, rivastigmine, donepezil hydrochloride and galantamine and memantine.

Tacrine was the first approved drug for dementia, introduced in 1993.

Symptomatic Management

Treatment of anxiety symptoms with benzodiazepines like lorazepam. Special care should be taken to prevent misuse and dependence. If psychotic symptoms are there, antipsychotic like haloperidol or risperidone can be given if essential. Antipsychotics are contraindicated in Lewy body dementia.

For depressive symptoms, small dose of selective serotonin reuptake inhibitors (SSRI) like citalopram is prescribed.

Short-term hospitalization is needed with aggravation of symptoms. Along with medical management, memory enhancement techniques in the early stages can prevent further deterioration.

Family education regarding illness, features, treatment, nursing care in home situation are important. Supportive services to the caregivers can also contribute more.

Prognosis

Prognosis of dementia is poor as it is a progressive disorder which is irreversible in nature. But some types like hypothyroid dementia are reversible, if identified and treated early. Early detection and treatment can prevent further progression of disease.

Differences between delirium and dementia are shown in Table 7.2.

Table 7.2: Differences between delirium and dementia

Delirium	*Dementia*
• Nature of onset is acute	• Onset is insidious
• Reversible/transient	• Usually irreversible
• Clouding of consciousness is there	• Consciousness not affected
• Disorientation present	• Disorientation in later stages only
• Immediate and recent memory affected	• Recent memory is affected
• Sleep-wake cycle grossly changed	• Usually normal
• Attention, concentration, comprehension are affected	• Affected as condition progress
• Perception affected—illusion and visual hallucination present	• Hallucinations present in later stage

ORGANIC AMNESTIC SYNDROME

It is the memory impairment due to organic cause; occur without severe alteration in consciousness and attention.

Clinical Features

- Severe impairment in recent memory (inability to learn new information/short-term memory impairment).

- Impairment in remote memory (inability to recall previously learned materials/long-term memory impairment).
- No global impairment in intellectual functions.
- Disorientation to time and place.
- Confabulation.

Etiology

Thiamine deficiency is the common cause of this, and occurs due to chronic alcoholism (Wernicke-Korsakoff syndrome).

Cerebrovascular disease, cerebral neoplasms, head injury and hypoxia are the other causes.

Transient amnestic syndrome may occur in epileptic seizures, after electroconvulsive therapy, severe migraine, and drug overdose.

NURSING MANAGEMENT OF ORGANIC MENTAL DISORDERS

Nursing Diagnosis	*Objectives*	*Plan of actions*
1. Risk for trauma related to disorientation/ confusion or muscular incoordination or perceptual disturbances—hallucination	Client will not experience any injury	• Assess the patient for disorientation and confusion • Ensure safety measures • Provide bed with siderails to prevent accidental falls • Provide low stimuli environment, by keeping the patient nearer to nurse's station or in ICU • Keep minimum furniture in room and arrange it properly to prevent accidental hit and falls • Observe patient's behaviors frequently and not leave him/her alone, assign staff on one-to-one basis if possible or keep relative with the patient • Accompany and assist client in ambulation, provide wheelchair while transporting for investigations • Provide safe environment, by keeping all harmful objects out of reach of patient • If the patient is restless, administer medications as per order • If all these measures fail, restraints can be used with order and specific precautions

Contd...

Contd...

Nursing Diagnosis	*Objectives*	*Plan of actions*
2. Risk for self-directed or other directed violence related to neurological dysfunction/delusions/ hallucinations/confusion/ substance intoxication	Client will maintain calm, with minimal agitated behavior	• Assess patient's behavior pattern—observe for agitation or increase in anxiety and passively monitor to avoid violence • Maintain a low stimuli environment with low noise, dim light and less number of people • Provide safe environment by keeping all dangerous objects out of reach of patient and help in preventing harm to self and to others • Maintain adequate number of staff in all shifts to manage, if patient become violent. This will ensure the safety of other patients and staff • Avoid arguments and shouting. Be supportive and maintain calm and quiet approach • Reorient to reality, if patient is confused or hallucinating • Administer tranquilizers and if needed use soft restraints in consultation with doctor • Teach the caregivers about early symptoms and management of violence
3. Disturbed sensory perception (specify), related to brain dysfunction (specify etiology), or substance intoxication/with-drawal evidenced by hallucinatory behavior (talking to self, laughing to self) or verbalization	Client maintains real perception and reality orientation	• Assess the nature and content of hallucination or other sensory problems • Maintain low stimuli environment with low noise and less people • Avoid reinforcement of hallucinations by avoiding over discussions on that and by focusing on reality. Tell the patient that you are not sharing that perception • Reorient the person frequently to the surroundings • Reassure and ensure safety if the patient shows fear and anxiety. Stay with the patient and talk about real matters

Contd...

Contd...

Nursing Diagnosis	*Objectives*	*Plan of actions*
		• without argument. Follow simple and clear language, as per the patient's level of understanding • Teach the caregivers about hallucinatory behavior and management of such problems
4. Self-care deficit (specify) related to cognitive impairment evidenced by inability to bath/groom/ feed	He/she maintains activities of daily living with assistance from the caregiver	• Assess the self-care ability of patient through observation and by asking • Provide assistance in self-care as per the need (specify) • Provide structured environment and use simple language to avoid confusion • Stay with the patient and give necessary guidance and support in self- care activities. Encourage independence by giving adequate time and by motivating the patient
5. Impaired verbal communication related to cognitive impairment, evidenced by disorientation and poor attention and irrelevant speech or absence of speech	Client communicates his/her basic needs and understands the interaction with primary caregivers and others	• Assess the communication problems in the patient • Anticipate and meet the needs of the patient. Consistency in caregivers—staff or family member will help in this • Encourage communication of the patient by validating and seeking clarification of his speech and gestures • Any effort for effective communication should be appreciated then and there Encourage eye to eye contact and face to face manner in communication
6. Imbalanced nutrition less than body requirement related to less intake and inability to feed by self- evidenced by loss of body weight, pallor, weakness	He/she maintains normal feeding by self or with assistance from caregiver	• Assess the feeding pattern and observe for features of malnutrition and dehydration • Encourage small frequent feeds as per patient's likes • Increase fluid intake to prevent dehydration • Provide high protein and energy rich foods (make changes as per

Contd...

Contd...

Nursing Diagnosis	*Objectives*	*Plan of actions*
		• patient's physical illness and medical advice) • Educate about balanced diet and cheap and locally available foods • Supplement vitamins and minerals if needed
7. Chronic confusion related to impairment in brain function evidenced by progressive cognitive impairment	He/she maintains oriented to the environment	• Assess the cognitive functioning of the client • Frequently reorient the client to reality by providing calendar and clock • Allow the client to use familiar things or own belongings • Plan daily routine and follow that Teach the caregiver about home care of the client by following planned schedule • Call him/her by name and give explanations clearly and in simple terms • Give positive feedback for any positive effort, as real perception and communication

CONCLUSION

Management of organic mental disorders usually begins in a casualty department. Once the acute phase is managed, they may be referred to psychiatry department. Ask for the general features of organic mental disorder, and specific clinical features. Once the diagnosis and underlying etiology is identified, treatment of specific etiology can reverse delirium or dementia (treatable dementia). Individualized nursing care can make improvement and will prevent complications.

BIBLIOGRAPHY

1. Ahuja N. A Short textbook of Psychiatry (Seventh edition). New Delhi: Jaypee Brothers Medical Publishers (P) Ltd, 2011.
2. Lalitha K. Mental Health and Psychiatric Nursing an Indian Perspective Bengaluru: VMG Book House, 2008.
3. Sadock BJ, Sadock VA, Ruiz P. Kaplan and Sadock's Synopsis of Psychiatry: Behavioral Sciences/Clinical Psychiatry (Ninth edition). Philadelphia: Wolters Kluwer, 2009.

4. Stuart GW, Laraia MT. Principles and Practice of Psychiatric Nursing. St. Louis: Mosby, 2001.
5. Townsend CM. Psychiatric Mental Health Nursing: Concepts of Care in Evidence-Based Practice (7th Edition). Philadelphia: FA Davis Company, 2012.
6. Vyas JN, Ghimire RS. Textbook of Postgraduate Psychiatry (Third edition). New Delhi: Jaypee Brothers Medical Publishers (P) Ltd, 2016.
7. World Health Organization. The ICD-10 Classification of Mental and Behavioral Disorders: Clinical Descriptions and Diagnostic Guidelines. Geneva: World Health Organization, 1992.

CHAPTER 8 Substance Use Disorder-Alcohol, Tobacco and Other Psychoactive Substance Use

INTRODUCTION

Psychoactive substances had been used by human for a very long time in order to enhance well-being and to reduce emotional discomfort. Use of psychoactive drugs often begins during adolescence and it produces physical, psychological problems and can often cause family dysfunctions.

TERMINOLOGIES USED

Drug

Refers to any substance which when taken by a living organism may modify one or more of its functions.

Psychoactive Substance

A drug that has effect on mental functioning.

Dependence

A state in which the intake of psychoactive substance takes on a high priority than other behaviors that had greater value and is characterized by physiological, behavioral and emotional responses.

Physical Dependence

Occurs when the person requires that particular drug so as to function normally, otherwise the person may experience symptoms.

Psychological Dependence

Occurs when the person requires the drug to maintain his thoughts, emotions and activities.

Tolerance

Increased dose of the drug is needed in order to produce the effects that were originally produced with lower dose.

Withdrawal

A state characterized by symptoms which occurs on total or partial stoppage of the drug, usually after repeated and high dose use.

Cross Tolerance

The ability of one drug to produce the effect of another drug, so that to prevent withdrawal symptoms.

PREVALENCE

The national household survey of drug use was the first systematic effort to document the nationwide prevalence of drug use in India. Alcohol (21.4%) was the primary substance used (apart from tobacco) followed by cannabis (3.0%) and opioids (0.7%).

National Family and Health Survey revealed an increase in alcohol use among males and an increase in tobacco use among women.

The drug abuse monitoring system evaluated the primary substance of abuse in inpatient treatment centers and found that the major substances were alcohol (43.9%), opioids (26%) and cannabis (11.6%).

ETIOLOGY (TABLE 8.1)

The etiology for psychoactive substance can be categorized as:

- Biological factors
- Psychological factors
- Social factors.

Table 8.1: Etiology for psychoactive substance use

Biological factors	*Psychological factors*	*Social factors*
• Genetic vulnerability • Personality disorders • Withdrawal effects • Biochemical factors	• Curiosity • Low self-esteem • Childhood trauma • Escape from reality • Early initiation of alcohol and tobacco • Poor stress management skills	• Peer pressure • Easy availability of drugs • Religious factors • Poor family support • Conflicts • Media

CLASSIFICATION

- F10 - Alcohol
- F11 - Opioids
- F12 - Cannabis
- F13 - Sedatives
- F14 - Cocaine

- F15 - Other stimulants
- F16 - Hallucinogens
- F17 - Tobacco
- F18 - Volatile solvents
- F19 - Multiple drugs

ALCOHOL

Alcoholism diagnosed as alcohol use disorder (DSM-5) is a state in which a person becomes physically and psychologically dependent on alcohol to the extent that he or she cannot function without it.

Effects of Alcoholism (Table 8.2)

Table 8.2: Effects of alcohol use

Short-term effects	*Long-term effects*	*Excessive use*
• Slurring of speech • Drowsiness • Emotional changes • Disturbed sleep • Euphoria • Flushing	• Pancreatitis • Cirrhosis • Tolerance	• Nausea and vomiting • Headache • Blackouts • Temporary loss of consciousness • Coma and death

Alcohol Use Disorder

According to DSM 5, alcohol use disorder is characterized by the presence of at least two of the following within 12 month period.

- Alcohol is taken in larger amounts or over an extended time.
- There is persistent desire or unsuccessful effort to cut down alcohol use.
- Great deal of time is spent in activities to obtain alcohol.
- Craving or a strong desire to take the drug.
- Recurrent alcohol use resulting in failure to fulfill the major role obligations at work, school.
- Important social, recreational and occupational activities are given up.
- Inability to control the desire to take the drug.
- Continue to take the drug in spite of the awareness regarding the harmful consequences of the drug.
- Tolerance.

Withdrawal Symptoms

Minor alcohol withdrawal symptoms like tremors, sweating, anxiety, nausea, vomiting, headache and insomnia often appear 6 to 12 hours after a person stops drinking. Persons may experience visual, auditory, or tactile hallucinations between 12 and 24 hours after they stop drinking. Three types of withdrawal symptoms are:

1. **Delirium tremens:** Occurs usually within 2–4 days after the complete stoppage of alcoholism. This is characterized by clouding of consciousness, disorientation, confusion, severe anxiety, visual hallucinations, profuse sweating ,seizures, hypertension, tachycardia, fever and dehydration. The classic triad of symptoms include clouding of consciousness, vivid hallucinations and tremor. The treatment of delirium tremens includes fluid and electrolyte replacement, thiamine supplementation and treatment of medical disorders.
2. **Alcoholic seizures:** Tonic-clonic seizures occur usually 12–48 hours after a heavy intake of alcoholism.
3. **Alcoholic hallucinosis:** This is characterized by the presence of auditory hallucinations during abstinence.

Treatment

The treatment approach used in alcoholism can be categorized as:

- **Detoxification:** The purpose of detoxification is symptomatic management of withdrawal symptoms. The drugs of choice are benzodiazepines. Chlordiazepoxide, lorazepam and diazepam are commonly used.
  Vitamin B (Thiamine) is usually administered parentally for 3–5 days to prevent Wernicke-Korsakoff psychosis. Thiamine is orally administered for at least 6 months. Adequate hydration is also ensured.
- **Treatment of alcohol dependence:** The important treatment measures include:
  - *Deterrent agents:* Disulfiram is the commonly used deterrent agent. When alcohol is taken, it is metabolized into acetaldehyde by the enzyme alcohol dehydrogenase, and acetaldehyde is further metabolized to acetate by aldehyde dehydrogenase. Disulfiram inhibits the action of aldehyde dehydrogenase, thereby causing the accumulation of acetaldehyde. When alcohol is taken with disulfiram, there will be increased accumulation of acetaldehyde. This produces disulfiram—ethanol reaction (DER) (Fig. 8.1), characterized by flushing, hypotension, nausea, vomiting and giddiness. Disulfiram-ethanol reaction sometimes produces life-threatening conditions like myocardial infarction, shock, convulsions and coma. Patient and the relatives should be taught about DER and that even small amount of alcohol intake can produce symptoms. The usual dose is 250–500 mg/

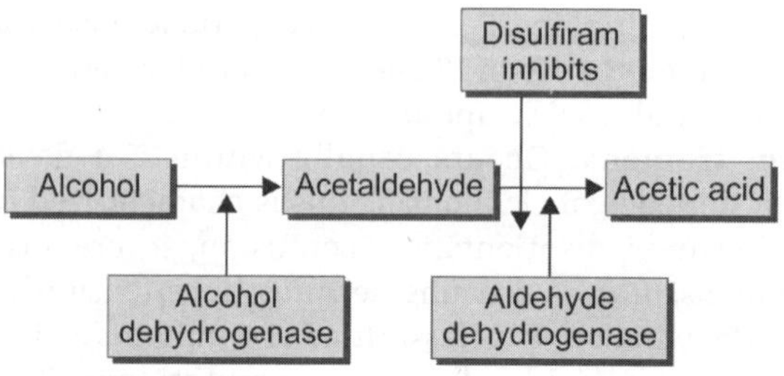

Fig. 8.1: Mechanism of action of disulfiram

day. Citrated calcium carbimide, metronidazole are also used as deterrent agents.

- *Anticraving agent:* Acamprosate and naltrexone are the commonly used anticraving agents.
- *Psychosocial therapies:* Behavior therapy, family therapy and group therapy are also used as treatment approach. In self-help groups such as Alcoholic Anonymous (AA), group members are allowed to share their experiences and they help each other. Alcoholic Anonymous is a nonprofessional, self-supporting and exist almost everywhere. There is no eligibility to be a member based on age or educational requirements. Membership is given to any person who desires to stop his or her drinking problem. Meetings are held frequently in which persons describe how they started alcoholism and their life after joining alcoholic anonymous.

Complications of Alcohol Dependence

Medical complications	*Social complication*
Gastrointestinal System • Peptic ulcer • Gastritis • Carcinoma of stomach, liver • Cirrhosis of liver • Hepatitis • Pancreatitis **Nervous System** • Peripheral neuropathy • Cerebellar degeneration • Head injury • Alcoholic dementia **Cardiovascular System** • Coronary artery disease • Cardiomyopathy	• Accidents • Marital conflicts • Divorce • Financial loss • Rape

OPIOIDS

There is a wide variety of opioids which are used by different routes—oral, injections or through nasal route.

Classification

The commonly used opioids can be classified as:
- **Natural opiates:** Morphine, codeine
- **Synthetic opioids:** Heroin, methadone

The opioids which mostly produce dependence are morphine and heroine. Heroine is available in an impure form known as brown sugar.

Opioid drugs also can cause euphoria, drowsiness, nausea, vomiting and constipation. Heroine when combined with alcohol can even cause death. When opioids are taken in large doses it can produce.

CLINICAL FEATURES OF OPIOID INTOXICATION AND WITHDRAWAL

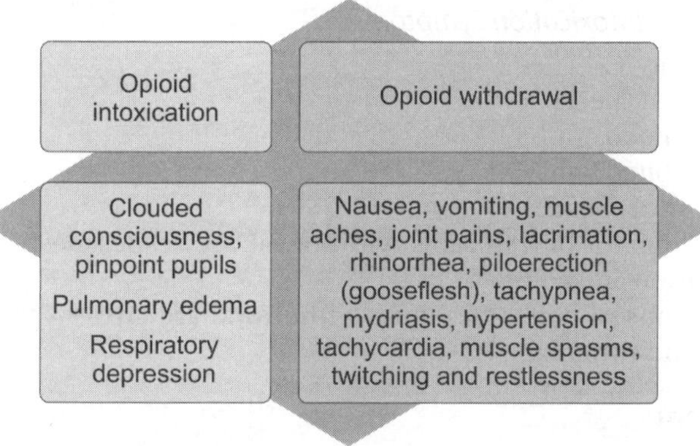

Fig. 8.2: Clinical features of opioid intoxication and withdrawal

Treatment

Narcotic antagonists (Naloxone, Naltrexone) are used when there is overdose of opioids. Methadone is used to reduce the withdrawal symptoms.

Psychotherapy, behavior therapy, family therapy, group therapy and motivational enhancement therapy are used.

CANNABIS

Cannabis is obtained from hemp plant. The ingredients are known as marijuana.

Effect of Cannabis

Intoxication

Characterized by impairment of consciousness, disorientation, tachycardia, photophobia, dry mouth and lacrimation. Depersonalization, derealization and visual hallucination are observed.

Treatment

Treatment is mainly based on symptoms. Psychotic symptoms are treated with antipsychotics.

SEDATIVES

These are drugs which decrease the functions of central nervous system. These are often referred to as Red Devil. They mainly include barbiturates and benzodiazepines.

Effect of Sedatives

Barbiturates Intoxication Symptoms

- Irritability
- Increased speech
- Labile mood
- Disinhibited behavior
- Slurring of speech.

Symptoms of barbiturates withdrawal are restlessness, tremors, hypertension and coma.

Symptoms of benzodiazepine withdrawal are anxiety, irritability, tremors and vomiting.

Treatment

Management of barbiturate intoxication includes induction of vomiting and gastric lavage. Supportive treatment should also to be initiated.

COCAINE

Cocaine is a weak alkaline compound which is a central stimulant. It is available in the nick name *Crack.*

Effects of Cocaine

Symptoms of cocaine intoxication are tactile hallucination (cocaine bugs), tachycardia, hypertension and labile mood.

Symptoms of cocaine withdrawal are vivid and unpleasant dreams, increased appetite, insomnia and psychomotor retardation or agitation.

Treatment

The treatment consists of oxygenation, muscle relaxants in case of cocaine overdose. Psychosocial therapies like behavior therapy and supportive therapy are effective to prevent relapse.

STIMULANTS

These are drugs which increase the function of central nervous system. Amphetamine is the most common stimulant drug.

Effect of Stimulant

Symptoms of amphetamine intoxication are tachycardia, hypertension, seizures, fever, tremors and ataxia.

Symptoms of amphetamine withdrawal are depression, apathy, fatigue hypersomnia and hyperphagia.

Treatment

Management measures for amphetamine intoxication are cold sponging, anticonvulsants and antihypertensives. Acidification of urine using ammonium chloride 500 mg helps in the elimination of amphetamines.

HALLUCINOGENS

Hallucinogens are a group of drugs that produce hallucinations. Hallucinogens can be classified into classic hallucinogens (LSD) and dissociative drugs (Phencyclidine).

Lysergic Acid Diethylamide (LSD) is a strong hallucinogen. Intoxication can produce depersonalization, derealization and illusions. Kaleidoscopic visual hallucinations are also experienced. Use of the drug produce a phenomenon called humanity identification in which the individual develops feelings of love and affection towards all persons. Flashbacks may also occur.

Treatment of acute intoxication includes administration of anxiolytics, antipsychotics and antidepressants.

Phencyclidine is an atypical hallucinogen. It is also called peace pill and angel dust. Intoxication can produce euphoria, agitation and sometimes delirium, stupor mania or depression may occur.

Treatment is by gastric lavage and administration of antipsychotics.

TOBACCO

Tobacco use may be defined as any habitual use of the tobacco plant leaf and its products. Tobacco contains nicotine, which is a psychoactive ingredient. Tobacco is mostly used by smoke inhalation of cigarettes, pipes, and cigars. *Smokeless tobacco* refers to a variety of tobacco products that are sniffed, sucked, or chewed. Tobacco cigarette smoking is the most common substance use disorder.

Smoking causes cancer, heart disease, stroke, lung diseases, diabetes and chronic obstructive pulmonary disease.

Tobacco Intoxication

Characterized by insomnia, bizarre dreams, lability of mood and impairment in functioning.

Tobacco Withdrawal State

Features include malaise, anxiety, insomnia, poor concentration and increased appetite.

VOLATILE SOLVENTS

Inhalant users inhale vapor or aerosol propellant gases using plastic bags held over the mouth or by breathing from a solvent-soaked rag or an open container.

Volatile Solvents Intoxication

Symptoms include apathy, lethargy, abusive nature and impairment in attention, memory and judgment.

NURSING MANAGEMENT

Nursing Care Plan (Table 8.3)

Table 8.3: Nursing care plan for clients with psychoactive substance use

Nursing diagnosis	*Objective*	*Plan of action*
Risk for self-directed injury related to depressed mood as evidenced by dangerous behavior.	Client will not harm self Client will seek out staff when he has suicidal ideation.	• Observe client's behavior frequently. • Observe for suicidal behaviors: Verbal statements, such as I am going to kill myself'. • Determine suicidal intent and available measures. • Obtain verbal or written contract that he agrees not to harm self or to seek out staff when such ideation occurs. • Provide safe environment for the client. • Encourage verbalizations of his feelings. • Maintain 1:1 nurse patient ratio. • Place client in room close to nurse's station.

Contd...

Contd...

Nursing diagnosis	*Objective*	*Plan of action*
		• Remove all harmful objects from client's reach (sharp objects, straps, belts, ties, glass items). • Observe closely during meals and medication administration. • Ask the patient not to lock the bathroom from inside.
Denial related to ineffective coping skills	Client verbalizes awareness of relationship of substance abuse to current situation. Client verbalize acceptance of responsibility for own behavior.	• Convey attitude of acceptance. • Clear the doubts honestly. • Provide information regarding the effects of drug use. • Remain nonjudgmental. • Observe for any changes in behavior (restlessness, increased psychomotor activity). • Provide positive feedback for expressing awareness of denial in self and others. • Maintain firm expectation that patients attend therapy groups regularly
Ineffective individual coping related to negative role modeling, inadequate support systems	Client identifies in-effective coping behaviors. Client use effective coping skills.	• Assess the client's perception of current situation. • Assess previous methods of coping with life's problems • Set limits on his behavior. • Encourage verbalization of feelings, fears and anxiety. • Explore alternative coping strategies. • Teach patient about the use of relaxation techniques. • Involve in diversional activity. • Encourage involvement with self-help groups (Alcoholics, Narcotics Anonymous). • Maintain a quiet and safe environment
Powerlessness related to extreme desire to take the drug	Client gain control over desire to take drug	• Help the client to recognize that he is not able to control his desire to take the drug. • Talk in a caring, nonjudgmental way how drug has affected life. • Involve patient in treatment plan. • Explore alternative solutions for coping with the problems. • Help the client in selecting most appropriate alternative decision.

Contd...

Contd...

Nursing diagnosis	*Objective*	*Plan of action*
		• Assist client to take the measures to enhance health and structure healthy diversion from drug use (maintaining a balanced diet, getting adequate rest, exercise and relaxation techniques).
Imbalanced nutrition less than body requirements related to inadequate dietary intake, poor appetite	Client demonstrates progressive weight gain. Client verbalizes awareness regarding effects of substance abuse, reduced dietary intake on nutritional status.	• Assess the patient's nutritional intake. • Assess weight and activity. • Instruct the client to take small and frequent feeds. • Provide opportunity to choose foods and snacks to meet dietary plan. • Consult with dietician.
Low self-esteem related to situational crisis, withdrawal from alcohol/other drugs	Identify feelings for negative perception of self. Verbalize an increased sense of self-worth.	• Encourage verbalization of client's feelings. • Discuss in a nonjudgmental way about patient's behavior and substance use. • Inform the client that substance use is the problem and that problems can be managed without the use of drugs. • Provide positive reinforcement for adaptive behavior. • Involve patient in group therapy. • Administer antipsychotic medications as prescribed.
Ineffective family process related to inadequate coping skills, lack of problem-solving skills	Participate in individual family programs.	• Determine the roles of family members and circumstances involving drug use. • Determine understanding of current situation and previous coping measures. • Encourage family members to be aware of their own feelings. Allow them to ventilate the feelings and thoughts related to drug use. • Provide information to patient and family about the effects of substance use on the family. • Encourage involvement with self-help groups—Alcoholics and Narcotics Anonymous, Al-Anon.

Contd...

Contd...

Nursing diagnosis	*Objective*	*Plan of action*
Knowledge deficient related to interference with learning	Client verbalizes awareness of disease condition, prognosis and complications. Client participates in treatment program including plan for follow-up/long-term care.	• Assess the knowledge regarding the disease condition. • Provide written and verbal information. • Inform relationship of drug use to current situation. • Educate about effects of specific drug(s) used. • Discuss the risk for emergence of withdrawal symptoms. • Provide information regarding variety of available organizations and programs for assistance and referral.

Prevention of Substance Use Disorders

Prevention of substance use disorders can be classified into 3 levels. They are:

1. **Primary prevention:** Mass campaigning can be conducted to spread the information regarding the ill effects of substance use disorders. Mass media, health exhibition for the public and school health programs can be arranged to disseminate the knowledge. Education given to the public should not only focus on improving the knowledge, but also change the attitude to quit substance use. Young people can be motivated to select a variety of alternatives to substance use, which include music, sports and games. Youth can also be taught social skills and assertive skills to overcome the peer pressure, which is one of the important contributing factor. Narcotics Control Bureau in India has launched programs to spread awareness to students, parents and teachers regarding the effects of drug abuse.
2. **Secondary prevention:** This includes early detection and prompt treatment of substance use disorders. Motivational counseling is usually given for those affected by this disorder.
3. **Tertiary prevention:** Prevention of disability arising out of substance use disorders and rehabilitation are addressed in tertiary prevention.

CONCLUSION

Substance use disorders are always a matter of major concern because of their impact on individual, family and society as a whole. Health education in schools, early treatment and rehabilitation of clients with substance use disorders, mass campaigning are some of the activities that can be undertaken to reduce the burden of substance use disorders.

BIBLIOGRAPHY

1. Ahuja N. A Short Textbook of Psychiatry (Seventh edition). New Delhi: Jaypee Brothers Medical Publishers (P) Ltd, 2011.
2. American Psychiatric Association. Diagnostic and Statistical Manual of Mental Disorders (5th ed). Washington DC, 2013.
3. Frisch N, Lawarence Frisch. Psychiatric Mental Health Nursing (Fourth Edition). Delmar Cengage Learning, New York, 2011.
4. Halter, Margaret J, Varcarolis, Elizabeth M (Eds). Varcarolis' Foundations of Psychiatric Mental Health Nursing: A Clinical Approach. St Louis, Mo: Elsevier, 2014.
5. Kapoor B. Textbook of Psychiatric Nursing. Delhi: Kumar Publishing House, 2014.
6. Narcotic Control Bureau. Available from: http://www.narcoticsindia.nic.in (Accessed on 2017 May).
7. National Family Health Survey India-3. Available from: http://www.nfhsindia.org/nfhs3.html (Accessed on 2017 March).
8. National Survey on the Extent, Pattern and Trends of Drug Abuse in India. Available from http://www.unodc.org/pdf/india/presentations/india_national_survey_2004.pdf (Accessed on 2017 May).
9. Sadock BJ, Sadock VA, Ruiz P. Kaplan and Sadock's Synopsis of Psychiatry: Behavioral Sciences/Clinical Psychiatry (Ninth edition). Philadelphia: Wolters Kluwer, 2009.
10. Schultz MJ, Videbeck LS. Lippincott's Manual of Psychiatric Nursing Care Plans. Philadelphia: Wolters Kluwer, 2012.
11. Sreevani R. A Guide to Mental Health and Psychiatric Nursing (Third Edition). New Delhi: Jaypee Brothers Medical Publishers (P) Ltd, 2016.
12. Theodore DD. Textbook of Mental Health Nursing. India: Elsevier, 2015.
13. Vyas JN, Ghimire RS. Textbook of Postgraduate Psychiatry (Third edition). New Delhi: Jaypee Brothers Medical Publishers (P) Ltd, 2016.
14. World Health Organization. The ICD-10 Classification of Mental and Behavioral Disorders: Clinical Descriptions and Diagnostic Guidelines. Geneva: World Health Organization, 1992.

CHAPTER 9

Schizophrenia, Schizotypal and Delusional Disorders

INTRODUCTION

Schizophrenia is a chronic debilitating psychiatric disorder with wide range of symptoms, physiological changes, etiologies and prognoses. It is one of the worst diseases affecting mankind. Though there is effective treatment for schizophrenia, most of these patients discontinue the treatment due to the distressing side effects or other factors. Worldwide prevalence of schizophrenia is 1%. Studies show that schizophrenia is a disease of biological cause or may be considered as a brain disease.

Definition

Schizophrenia is a syndrome characterized by disordered thought, emotion and perception that are manifested as abnormal behavior and impairment in social competency.

In schizophrenia, the individual's thought will be strange and incoherent, and may loss the touch with the reality. They will be unable to manage their feelings and to maintain social relations.

Age of onset is usually in the late teens and young adulthood. Nature of onset may be either abrupt or insidious. Only 10–15% of cases have occurrence after the age of 45 years.

Historical Background

- Emil Kraepelin (1896) identified major psychiatric illness as two types: (i) Dementia praecox (which include paranoia, catatonia and hebephrenic) and (ii) Manic depressive illness.
- Eugen Bleuler (1911) coined the name schizophrenia (means 'splitting of mind') for Dementia praecox. He explained it as a group of disorders and called 'a group of schizophrenias'. He explained the fundamental symptoms of schizophrenia (also known as Bleuler's 4 A's) and accessory symptoms as delusions, hallucinations and negativism.
- Kurt Schneider (1959) pointed out some symptoms (Schneider's First Rank Symptoms—SFRS), that help in the diagnosis of schizophrenia. But it is not specific for it, and may be seen in mood disorders and organic mental disorders. He explained second rank symptoms of schizophrenia also, but they are less important for diagnosis.

Epidemiology

- Worldwide prevalence of schizophrenia is 1%.
- According to WHO report 2001 (mental health report 2001), about 24 million people worldwide suffer from schizophrenia. The point of prevalence of schizophrenia is 0.5–1%.
- The incidence of schizophrenia is 0.5/1,000 population. The incidence varies from 7–16 cases per lakh population and it will vary from country to country.
- About 3–4/1,000 in every community suffer from schizophrenia. Only 1% of general population is at risk of developing this disease in their lifetime.
- Prevalence is equal in both sexes. But onset is later (25–35 years) in females as compared to that of males (15–25 years). Two-third of the cases belong to the age group of 15–30 years.
- Previously it was believed that this disease belonged to low socioeconomic status. But now it is common in people with high socioeconomic status and urban areas.

ICD Classification

F20 – F29	**:**	**Schizophrenia, schizotypal and delusional disorders**
F20	:	Schizophrenia
F20.0	:	Paranoid schizophrenia
F20.1	:	Hebephrenic schizophrenia
F20.2	:	Catatonic schizophrenia
F20.3	:	Undifferentiated schizophrenia
F20.4	:	Post-schizophrenic depression
F20.5	:	Residual schizophrenia
F20.6	:	Simple schizophrenia
F21	:	Schizotypal disorders
F22	:	Delusional disorders

ETIOLOGY OF SCHIZOPHRENIA

Like other mental disorders, we cannot point out a single cause for schizophrenia. There is a combination of biopsychosocial factors that contribute to development of the disorder.

Etiology of schizophrenia, though not clear, there are many theories that support the biopsychosocial factors.

A. Biological Theories

Genetic Hypothesis

It points out about the chance of occurrence of schizophrenia, if there is a positive family history. Hypothesis says that there is 10% chance for developing schizophrenia, if a first degree relative is affected.

- 40%—if both the parents are affected
- 14%—if one parent has the illness
- 8%—if one sibling is affected
- 47% chance in case of monozygotic twins.

Brain Pathology

Some pathological changes occur in brain. They are:

- Loss of grey matter
- Hypofrontality or abnormal neuronal migration leading to impairment in frontal lobe functions
- Mild cortical atrophy
- Shrinkage of cerebellar vermis
- Thickening of Corpus callosum.

Biochemical Theories

It explains about the dysregulation of neurotransmitters in brain as etiology.

- **Dopamine hypothesis:** It says that there is a functional increase in dopamine in the postsynaptic receptors and psychotic features are caused by excess of dopamine.
- Dysregulation of serotonin, Gamma Amino Butyric Acid (GABA) and Acetylcholine.
  Dysregulation of serotonin causes positive and negative symptoms.

There is loss of GABA in neurons that lead to hyperactivity of dopaminergic neurons in brain.

B. Psychological Theories

These theories explain about the psychological aspects that can add the risk of schizophrenia:

- **Stress-vulnerability hypothesis:** It says that schizophrenia is precipitated by or triggered by stressful situations. Many stressful events are seen before the onset/relapse of schizophrenia. Increased Expressed Emotions (EE) of significant others in the family can lead to early relapse.
- **Family Theories:** It points out the role of faulty family situations. Several theories are proposed based on family, and the major facts in these are:
  - *'Schizophrenogenic mothers,' Lack of real parents, maternal deprivation or anxious mother*—All these factors will lead to lack of effective mother child relationship and may lead to poor socialization or social withdrawal of the child.
  - *Marital schism or skew*—Marital schism is severe chronic disequilibrium and discord among parents. But in marital skew, relative equilibrium is achieved, but family life is distorted.

- *Double bind theory:* Double bind is an emotionally distressing dilemma in communication in which an individual receives two or more conflicting messages. Theory says that schizophrenic thinking may not be an inborn mental disorder, but a learned confusion in thinking.
- *Expressed emotions (EE):* High expressed emotions (hostility, critical comments, emotional over involvement of significant others) in the family contract to relapse.

- **Psychoanalytic Theory:** It explains impaired ego functioning. Theory explains that there is regression to preoral and oral stage of psychosexual development with over use of denial, projection and reaction formation. This leads to loss of touch with the reality.

C. Sociocultural Theories

It points out that schizophrenia is more common in people of lower socioeconomic status in the urban areas. Child who is deprived of love and affection from parents, alongwith lack of schooling, socialization and hard work/struggle for life leads to frustrations and anger.

D. Miscellaneous Theories

These are organic theories and include:

- **Viral hypothesis:** It says that schizophrenia is the result of an early brain insult due to viral infections. This affects brain development (changes in hippocampal cells occur in second trimester of pregnancy).
- **Autoimmune factors in schizophrenia:** Autoimmune diseases and frequent infections that require hospitalization are risk factors for schizophrenia. Brain reactive autoantibodies are the underlying mechanism here (Table 9.1).

Table 9.1: Etiological factors in schizophrenia

Biological Factors	
• Genetic factors	Presence of illness in the family is a risk for developing it – first degree relative – 10% – one parent – 14% – Both the parents—40%
• Brain pathology	Changes in brain-Grey matter loss – Enlarged ventricles – Mild cortical atrophy – Hypofrontality and impaired frontal function – Shrinkage of cerebellar vermis and thickening of corpus callosum

Contd..

Contd..

• Biochemical change	Functional increase in dopamine in postsynaptic receptor site Dysregulation in serotonin, Gamma aminobutyric acid (GABA) and acetylcholine
Psychological	
• Stress vulnerability	Stressors can precipitate or trigger
• Faulty family process	Marital schism and marital skew
• Communication deviance	Double bind communication
• Psychological development	Regression, over use of faulty mental mechanisms
Sociocultural	Low socioeconomic status
Miscellaneous	Viral hypothesis Autoimmune factors Birth and pregnancy

Clinical Features

Symptoms may be of sudden or gradual onset. Before the first episode, insomnia, inability to concentrate, tension, withdrawal or cognitive deficit may be there.

Clinical features are classified under different headings.

Bleulers 4 A's (Primary Symptoms)

- **Affective disturbances:** Inappropriate, blunted or flattened affect.
- **Autistic thinking:** Individual is unable to keep in touch with others and environment (withdrawal into self).
- **Ambivalence:** Inability to decide due to simultaneous occurrence of contradictory ideas, emotions, attitudes or desires in towards a person, thing or situation.
- **Associative disturbance:** Loosening of association in thought and speech. It is due to the inability to think logically. Thoughts are of unrelated topics.

Schneider's First Rank Symptoms (SFRS)

- **Audible thoughts or thought echo:** Hearing own thoughts as spoken aloud.
- **Hallucinatory voices (3rd persons):** Two or more persons/voices discussing the subject in third person or voices heard arguing or statement or reply. Hallucinating voices in the form of commenting one's action or in the form of running commentary.
- **Thought withdrawal:** Subject experience that thought are removed from his/her mind by an external force.
- **Thought insertion:** Subject experience that thoughts are imposed to his/her mind by some external force.

- **Thought broadcasting or thought diffusion:** Subject experience that thoughts are being escaped and people around are experiencing it.
- **Delusional perceptions:** Individual gives a personal and illogical meaning to a normal perception.
- **Somatic passivity:** Bodily sensations are experienced as being imposed by some external force.
- **Made feelings, made impulses and made volition or acts:** Individual experiences that his feelings, impulses and acts are under the control of some external force.

Positive Symptoms and Negative Symptoms

Positive Symptoms

- **Delusions:** Delusions of control, paranoid (persecutory), reference, infidelity, thought broadcast also.
- **Hallucinations:** Auditory and visual are common.
- **Disorganized speech and thinking:** Loosening of association, tangentiality, incoherence.
- **Disorganized behavior:** This includes lack of goal directed behavior, unpredictable, agitated behavior, silly/disinhibited/bizarre behavior. These activities are prompted by delusions and hallucinations.
- **Catatonic behavior:** It is the motor manifestation that may occur in two forms. Catatonic excitement and stupor.
- Other symptoms include depersonalization, derealization and somatic problems.

Negative Symptoms

- Affective flattening or blunting
- Alogia—lack of speech output
- Avolition—lack of initiation
- Anhedonia—inability to experience pleasure
- Attention impairment
- Asociality.

Thought and Speech Disorders

- **Autistic thinking:** Most classical feature of schizophrenia. Removing the person totally from the reality by preoccupation with own illogical rules.
- **Loosening of association:** It is the speech pattern which lack meaningful relationship with each other. In severe form of loosening, speech becomes incomprehensible and is known as incoherence.

- **Thought blocking:** It is one of the characteristic features of schizophrenia. There is sudden blockade of stream of speech before the thought is completed. Can occur with thought withdrawal.
- **Neologism:** Newly coined words or phrases that are not familiar to others. Sometimes normal words are used in a distorted way but the word derivation can be understood even if bizarre. These are called word approximation or paraphrasi, e.g. describing stomach as food vessel.
- **Delusions of different type:** Paranoid or persecutory delusions, delusion of reference, grandiose delusions, nihilistic delusions, somatic delusion and bizarre delusions.

As the part of speech disorder: Patient may show complete mutism (no speech production) as seen in stupor.

- **Poverty of speech** (decreased speech production).
- **Poverty of ideations** (speech amount is adequate, but content conveys little information).
- **Echolalia:** Repetition of words of the examiner.
- **Preservation:** Repetition of words beyond the point of relevance.
- **Verbigeration:** Senseless repetition of words or phrases.

Other thought problems are:

- Over inclusions—including irrelevant items in speech
- Impaired abstractions
- Ambivalence.

Disorders of Perception

- Hallucination—auditory hallucination
- Elementary and hallucination—hearing simple sounds rather than voices
- Thought echo—audible thoughts
- Third person hallucination
- Voices commenting one's own actions
- Only third person hallucinations are believed to be characteristics of schizophrenia
- Visual hallucination can also occur with auditory
- Tactile, gustatory and olfactory are least common.

Disorders of affect: Apathy, blunted affect, emotional shallowness, anhedonia, inappropriate emotional response.

Disorders of Motor Behavior

Either decrease spontaneity, inertia, stupor or increases in psychomotor activity (excitement, aggressions, restlessness and agitation, mannerisms, grimacing, stereotypic repetitive strange behavior) decreased self-care and poor grooming are common features. Catatonic features in catatonic schizophrenia.

- Poor facial expression with verbal or nonverbal communication.
- Negative symptoms also occur as the result of disorders of motor behavior.

Other associated features are:

- Poor occupational functioning
- Poor social relations and self-care
- Multiple somatic symptoms especially in early stages
- Insight is absent and social judgment is poor
- No problems with consciousness, orientation, attention, memory and intelligence
- There is no underlying organic cause
- There is no mood disorders
- Symptomatology changes overtime.

Suicide in Schizophrenia

The following problems in schizophrenia can lead to suicide:

- Co-morbid depressive symptoms
- Command hallucination
- Impulsive behavior
- Presence of anhedonia
- Return of insight.

TYPES OF SCHIZOPHRENIA

Clinical types of schizophrenia are (Table 9.2):

- Paranoid
- Disorganized or hebephrenic
- Catatonic
- Residual
- Undifferentiated
- Simple
- Postschizophrenic depression.

Table 9.2: Types of schizophrenia and the specific features

1. Paranoid schizophrenia	• Delusion—delusions of persecution, reference, grandiosity, control, infidelity • Hallucination—auditory, olfactory, gustatory hallucinations • Disturbed affect, speech and motor behavior • Guarded or reserved nature on mental status examination (MSE). Sometimes suspicious, hostile or aggressive • Occurrence is between 30–40 years

Contd..

Contd..

2. Hebephrenic schizophrenia	• Incoherent or disorganized speech and thought Loosening of association, word salad Disorganized behavior • Uninhibited, purposeless and regressive or primitive behavior. • Distortion of reality with delusions or hallucinations • Emotional disturbances—Flattened or inappropriate affect, giggling, mirror gazing • Poor hygiene and self-care due to avolition • Social withdrawal • Onset is in early 20's • Severe deterioration, disintegration of personality with worst prognosis
3. Catatonic schizophrenia	Motor disturbance is marked and occur in two forms: 1. **Catatonic stupor:** Patient is responsive to environmental stimuli (stupor stage), remain immobile with rigid posture, waxy flexibility, mutism, negativism/refuses to respond. 2. **Catatonic excitement:** Looks excited due to excess movement i.e. purposeless, bizarre or unusual, stereotyped movements or assume very strange or inappropriate stance, senseless mimicking of words or movements of others (echolalia and echopraxia) mannerisms and grimacing
4. Residual schizophrenia	• Prominent negative symptoms—under activity, lack of speech, poor eye contact, avolition and poor self-care • Illogical thinking • Psychotic features—delusions and hallucinations are not prominent • There will be history of at least one episode of schizophrenia in the past with a period of 1 year • Absence of dementia or organic cause
5. Undifferentiated type	• Common type • Criteria for schizophrenia will be there, but features are not of single subtype of schizophrenia
6. Simple schizophrenia	• Early onset with slow progressive nature—early features are loss of interest and being aimless, socially withdrawn. So the personal behavior seems to be indifferent • Negative symptoms—apathy, under activity, lack of initiation, poor speech and nonverbal communication • Delusions and hallucination absent • Difficult to diagnose and prognosis is poor
7. Postschizophrenic depression	• Depressive symptoms or depressive episode that arise in the aftermath of schizophrenia with low level schizophrenia symptoms also • Usually occur 12 months after schizophrenia and risk for suicide is more in this period

Diagnosis

A detailed psychiatric history, mental status examination and observation helps in the diagnosis and in differentiating it from mood disorders and substance-induced psychosis.

Some investigations may be needed to rule out physical disorders as thyroid problems, renal or hepatic dysfunctions, vitamin deficiencies.

Radio diagnostic studies like CT Scan and MRI will rule out the underlying neurologic problems.

Some neuroanatomical changes like widening of sulci, enlarged ventricles and cerebellar atrophy are some suggestive features of schizophrenia. But these are not used in clinical practice. ICD10 criteria is widely accepted as the basis for diagnosis.

TREATMENT

Biological Therapies

Pharmacotherapy

Acute phase of schizophrenia is managed with antipsychotics. Typical or conventional antipsychotics are used in management of positive symptoms, especially in case of aggression. It is not given on a regular basis due to its adverse effects.

Chlorpromazine and haloperidol are the commonly used drugs of this group. Long acting depot preparations like fluphenazine deconoate are used in noncompliant patients.

Now atypical antipsychotics are preferred due to their effect on wide range of signs and symptoms and less side effects. These are effective against mood symptoms also.

Commonly atypical antipsychotics are—clozapine, risperidone, olanzapine, quetiapine, ziprasidone, and aripiprazole.

Electroconvulsive Therapy (ECT)

Electroconvulsive Therapy is used in treatment of catatonic stupor, catatonic excitement, schizophrenia that are not responding to drugs or other therapies. Patients who experience severe side effects also can be treated with ECT.

Psychosocial Therapies

- Family therapy
- Group therapy
- Cognitive therapy
- Social skill training
- Milieu therapy.

Along with treatment measures, psychosocial rehabilitation services can be provided once the acute phase is over or based on the patient's interests and capability.

They must be guided in utilizing the available services and community support groups.

PROGNOSIS

Factors that indicate good prognosis include:
- Acute or abrupt onset indicate good prognosis
- Later age of onset
- Good premorbid personality
- Presence of precipitating factor and short duration of illness
- Dominance of positive symptoms
- Good social support
- Married people
- Female gender.

NURSING MANAGEMENT

Table 9.3: Nursing care plan

Nursing Diagnosis	*Objectives*	*Plan of actions*
1. Disturbed thought process related to biochemical changes/inability to trust (as evidenced by extreme suspiciousness/ impaired volition, inability to concentrate, or solve problems)	He/she remains free of delusional thinking	• Assess the nature and content of delusion • Do not argue or deny the belief, but indicate that you do not share the belief. Discourage over discussions on it • Reinforce and focus on reality. Talk about real things • Maintain assertive, matter of fact, but genuine approach • Reassure the patient and family with calm and quiet approach and acceptance • Give positive reinforcement for realistic thoughts and behavior • Administer antipsychotics as per the order **For Suspicious Patients** • Promote development of trust, by assigning same staff and by being honest • Avoid physical contact or touch because they may perceive it as threatening and may respond violently • Avoid laughing and whispering or talking quietly as it can add the suspicion

Contd...

Contd...

Nursing Diagnosis	*Objectives*	*Plan of actions*
		• Serve food from a common container, sit and eat together to avoid fear of being poisoned • Mouth check should be done with each medication because they may spit it out • One-to-one interaction will be best. Avoid competitive activities • Maintain assertive, genuine and professional approach in care
2. Risk for violence—self-directed or other directed related to catatonic excitement, command, hallucinations, aggressive acts, active aggressive suicidal acts	He/she will not harm self/ others	• Maintain an environment with low level of stimulus • Observe client's behavior frequently to ensure safety • Remove all dangerous objects from environment (glass materials, sharp instruments, long clothes, chemicals and drugs) • Maintain a calm and quiet attitude towards client. Do not shout or argue with the client • Have sufficient staff available in each shift • Try to calm down him/her by gentle, firm talk. If necessary, drugs can be given • If all these measures fails, mechanical restraints can be used as last resort
3. Disturbed sensory perception related to biochemical changes (as evidenced by hallucinatory behavior—talking to self/ laughing to self)	Patient maintains normal perception	• Observe the client for signs of hallucinations • Convey an attitude of acceptance and encourage to share the content • Do not reinforce hallucinations. Say that you are not hearing it • Help the client to understand the link between hallucinations and anxiety • Try to distract the client from hallucination by calling name or other way • Talk about real matters. Avoid over discussions on hallucination because discussions may reinforce the hallucination

Contd...

Contd...

Nursing Diagnosis	*Objectives*	*Plan of actions*
		• Provide a planned routine for the patient so that they can be distracted • Administer antipsychotics as per the order
4. Impaired verbal communication related to disturbance in stream and form of thought (evidenced by loosening of association, word salad, clang association, echolalia, neologism)	He/she communicates effectively	• Maintain consistency in staff assignment to facilitate trust • Follow non-threatening approach • Anticipate and fulfill client's needs till functional communication has been established • Orient the client to reality by calling his/her name and validate his/her communication • Explain matters in simple, clear language and should be as per the level of understanding of client • Correlate both verbal and nonverbal responses meaningfully • Give positive reinforcement for effective communication
5. Social isolation related to withdrawal into self/suspiciousness/preoccupation with thought (evidenced by dull affect, expression of aloneness imposed by others)	Patient shows effort to socialize	• Assess the interaction pattern and socialization of the client • Convey acceptance by being honest and by being an active listener. This can add his/her self-esteem • Start with one-to-one interaction and gradually introduce to small groups • Encourage patient to communicate and give positive reinforcement for patient's effort for socialization • Help in maintenance of hygiene and grooming that can improve client's self esteem

Contd...

Contd...

Nursing Diagnosis	*Objectives*	*Plan of actions*
6. Disabled family coping related to lack of knowledge (evidenced by neglectful care of client with respect to human needs or illness/ treatment, by extreme denial or prolonged over concern, depression, hostility or aggression)	Family effectively cope up with the patient's behavior and cares with acceptance	• Assess the family's attitude to patient and his/her illness and the care aspects • Educate family members about etiology, signs and symptoms, need for long-term treatment • Educate the caregivers about drug therapy, special care for the specific drugs and side effects • Advise caregivers to avoid expressed emotions while caring these patients • Encourage family members to involve the patient in homely activities and social functions as far as possible • Plan and provide a schedule for daily activities. Ensure adequate sleep and rest, recreation, physical activities, reading, writing and in vocational training based on the capability

SCHIZOTYPAL DISORDER

Schizotypal disorder is a mental disorder with severe social anxiety, paranoia and unconventional beliefs. They feel discomfort in maintaining close relationship with people.

They think that others may harbor negative thoughts towards them, so will avoid others. Speech mannerisms and strange dressing pattern are also seen.

Definition: It is a disorder characterized by eccentric behavior and anomalies of thinking and affect which resemble those seen in schizophrenia.

Features are:

- Inappropriate or constricted affect
- Odd and eccentric behavior
- Social withdrawal
- Magical thinking or odd believes
- Paranoid ideas
- Obsessive ruminations
- Illusions, depersonalization or derealization, auditory hallucinations
- Occasional transient quasy-psychotic episode.

Schizotypal disorder occurrs approximately in 3% of the general population and is more common in males.

Management

- Usually treated with low doses of antipsychotics.
- Antidepressants like SSRI (sertraline) also is effective especially if there is obsessive-compulsive features.
- Psychotherapy is not much effective.

DELUSIONAL DISORDER

Delusional disorders are mental disorders in which the patient presents with delusions but with no accompanying hallucinations, thought disorder, mood disorder and flattening of affect. Here delusions are not due to drugs or an underlying physical disorder.

Features are:

- Patient express delusions and these ideas influence his/her life very much.
- Person is very sensitive and humorless.
- Irritability and hostility or strong emotional reactions when opposes this delusion.
- It occurs as a primary disorder, chronic and mostly lifelong.
- No disturbance in general behavior.
- Individual experience an increased feeling of self-reference.

Etiology

No definite etiology, but genetic, biochemical and environmental factors have some role.

Management

Antipsychotics are not much effective in treating the primary delusion. Drug therapy is difficult due to the lack of insight in these persons.

Individual psychotherapy is helpful. Cognitive therapy, supportive psychotherapy are highly effective.

CONCLUSION

Schizophrenia is the most debilitating mental disorder and 50% of the beds in a psychiatric hospital is occupied by these patients. Good knowledge about the disorder—etiology, clinical features, treatment especially psychopharmacology and nursing care are very important. This will help in caring the patient and also in educating the caregivers and the public. Correlating this theoretical aspects with clinical practice will improve the quality of care and may help in better prognosis.

BIBLIOGRAPHY

1. Ahuja N. A Short Textbook of Psychiatry (Seventh edition). New Delhi: Jaypee Brothers Medical Publishers (P) Ltd, 2011.
2. Fontaine KL. Mental Health Nursing (Fifth edition). New Delhi: Pearson Education, 2009.
3. Kapoor B. Textbook of Psychiatric Nursing. Delhi: Kumar Publishing House, 2014.
4. Sadock BJ, Sadock VA, Ruiz P. Kaplan and Sadock's Synopsis of Psychiatry: Behavioral Sciences/Clinical Psychiatry (Ninth edition). Philadelphia: Wolters Kluwer, 2009.
5. Sreevani R. Psychology for Nurses (Second Edition). New Delhi: Jaypee Brothers Medical Publishers (P) Ltd, 2013.
6. Stuart GW, Laraia MT. Principles and Practice of Psychiatric Nursing. St Louis: Mosby, 2001.
7. Townsend CM. Psychiatric Mental Health Nursing: Concepts of Care in Evidence-Based Practice (7th Edition). Philadelphia: FA Davis Company, 2012.
8. Vyas JN, Ghimire RS. Textbook of Postgraduate Psychiatry (Third edition). New Delhi: Jaypee Brothers Medical Publishers (P) Ltd, 2016.

CHAPTER 10

Mood (Affective) Disorders

Human beings experience a wide range of emotions like sadness, happy, anger and anxious. Mood is defined as pervasive and sustained emotional response that can color the person's perception of the world. Affect is defined as a pattern of observable behavior associated with subjective feelings such as facial expression, tone of voice and gestures (Table 10.1).

Table 10.1: Difference between mood and affect

Characteristics	*Mood*	*Affect*
Assessment	Subjective	Objective
Definition	Pervasive and sustained emotional response	Immediate emotional response associated with ideas or image.
Emotions	Sadness, anxious, fear, happy	Normal, constricted, blunted and flat

DEFINITION

Mood disorders are disorders in which disturbance in mood is the predominant feature along with problems associated with social, psychomotor and cognitive functions. The word *mania* is derived from the Greek word mania meaning *madness.*

EPIDEMIOLOGY OF MOOD DISORDERS

- **Sex:** The incidence of bipolar mood disorders in male/female is equal. But depressive disorder is more common among females.
- **Age:** Majority develops bipolar disorders around the age of 30 and depressive disorders develop around 40 years.
- **Social class:** Occurs more among persons with high social class.
- **Marital status:** Bipolar mood disorders are more among unmarried and divorced individuals.
- **Occupation:** Professionals are more affected than non-professionals.

ETIOLOGY OF MOOD DISORDER

Etiology of mood disorders can be categorized into biological, psychological and social factors.

- **Biological theories:**
  - *Genetic hypothesis:* Genetic factors play an important role in the causation of mood disorders. If one parent has bipolar disorder, the life time risk for their child is 25–27% and if both parents are affected, the risk is 50–75%. Concordance rate in mood disorders is 65% for monozygotic twins and 20% for dizygotic twins.
  - *Biochemical theories:* Dysfunction of certain neurotransmitters in the brain is postulated for the etiology of mood disorders. In mania, there is increase in monoamines—dopamine, serotonin and norepinephrine. Increased norepinephrine accounts for the aggressive behavior. Increased dopamine is responsible for the psychotic features and hyperactivity. Deficit in the activity of gamma-aminobutyric acid (GABA) explains the etiology of mania.
  - *Neurophysiological hypothesis:* Excitatory functions of neurons causes mania.
  - *Neuroanatomical changes:* Ventricular dilatation, changes in metabolism and blood flow in prefrontal cortex has been evident in brain imaging studies of patients with mood disorders.
- **Psychosocial theories:**
  - *Psychoanalytic theory:* According to psychoanalytic theory, mania is the result of use of reaction formation.
  - *Stress:* Stressful life events often act as a precipitating factor for the onset or relapse of mood disorders.

Classification of Mood Disorders (F30–F39)

- F30 - Manic episode
- F31 - Bipolar Mood Disorder (BPMD)
- F32 - Depressive episode
- F33 - Recurrent Depressive Disorder (RDD)
- F34 - Persistent mood disorder
- F38 - Other mood disorders
- F39 - Unspecified mood disorder

Manic Episode

Manic episode is characterized by an abnormal and persistently elevated, expansive or irritable mood lasting for at least 1 week and significantly impairing social or occupational functioning.

Clinical Features

Clinical features of manic episode are:

- **Elevated, expansible or irritable mood**
  Stages of elevated mood are:
  - *Euphoria:* Mild elevation of mood, increased psychological well-being.
  - *Elation:* Moderate elevation of mood, feeling of enjoyment and increased psychomotor activity.
  - *Exaltation:* Severe elevation of mood associated with delusion of grandeur.
  - *Ecstasy:* Very severe elevation of mood, intense sense of blissfulness.
- **Psychomotor activity:** Psychomotor activity is increased which ranges from restlessness to manic excitement. Patients often engage in goal directed activity. Manic stupor is also rarely seen.
- **Speech and thought:** Patient will be very talkative. There will be pressured speech, punning (using a same word with second meaning) and rhyming. Flight of ideas and incoherent speech will be present. Delusions of grandeur and persecution may develop. Patient will not be able to concentrate, distractibility present.
- **Goal directed activity:** Patient tries to do many tasks at a time. Often persistent hyperactivity leads to physical exhaustion. There will be increased social interaction even with strangers. They may engage in high-risk activities and have disinhibited behavior.
- **Other features:** Manic patients present with insomnia and decreased food intake. Insight is absent. Sexual desires are increased.

Types of Mania (Table 10.2)

Table 10.2: Characteristics features of hypomania, acute mania and delirious mania

Features	*Hypomania*	*Acute mania*	*Delirious mania*
Definition	Mild form of mania	Mania without psychotic features	Severe form of mania with psychotic features
Clinical Features			
Mood	Cheerful and mild elevation of mood	Moderate elevation of mood	Severe elevation of mood
Delusions	Usually absent	Grandiose ideas	Grandiose delusions Delusions of persecution

Contd...

Contd...

Features	*Hypomania*	*Acute mania*	*Delirious mania*
Hallucinations	Usually absent	Usually absent	Usually present
Cognition and perception	Attention and concentration may be impaired	Attention and concentration is impaired	Attention and concentration is severely impaired
Behavior and activity	Increased sociability, speech, over-familiarity, increased sexual energy and insomnia	Over activity, inappropriate behavior, pressured speech	Incomprehensible speech Aggressive or violent behavior

Management

- **Psychopharmacology**
  - *Mood stabilizers:* Lithium is the drug of choice for the treatment of acute manic episode. It is used for the prevention of recurrent manic episodes. The usual dose of lithium is 900–1500 mg. Regular monitoring of lithium therapy is required.
    - Therapeutic S. Lithium—0.8–1.2 mEq/L
    - Prophylactic S. Lithium—0.6–1.2 mEq/L
    - The serum lithium of more than 2 mEq/L indicates lithium toxicity.
    - Sodium valproate, carbamazepine and oxcarbamazepine are used for the treatment of mania.
  - *Antipsychotics:* Antipsychotics like Clozapine are used for the management of psychotic symptoms.
  - *Anxiolytics:* Benzodiazepines are used either alone or along with antipsychotics in reducing agitation. Lorazepam is particularly useful.
- **Electroconvulsive therapy (ECT):** ECT is not considered as the first line management of manic episode. It is used for those with delirious mania and neuroleptic malignant syndrome.
- **Psychosocial therapies:** Psychosocial therapies are used to increase the social, occupational and interpersonal functions. The psychosocial therapies effective in manic episode are psychoeducation, cognitive behavior therapy and group therapy.

Nursing Management (Table 10.3)

Table 10.3: Nursing care plan for a client with mania

Nursing diagnosis	*Objective*	*Plan of action*
Risk for other directed violence related to biochemical imbalances, threatened or actual aggression toward others	Client will not harm others	Assess the psychomotor activity of the client Provide a safe environment Set limits on behavior that is destructive or adversely affects others Reduce environmental stimuli Provide a consistent, structured environment Set realistic goals Give simple direct explanations (e.g. for procedures) Do not argue with the client Encourage the client to verbalize feelings such as anxiety and anger Explore ways to relieve tension with the client as soon as possible Provide physical activity under supervision Provide high calorie fluids (milk) Redirect the agitation and violent behavior to less dangerous activity (punching bag) Administer sedatives as prescribed
Imbalanced nutrition less than body requirements related to inadequate dietary intake, poor appetite	Client maintains optimum nutrition	Assess the nutritional status of the client Monitor the client's dietary pattern Provide finger foods that the client can carry with him or her (fortified milkshakes, sandwiches) Consider the likes and dislikes of the client. Frequently remind client to drink: 'Take two more sips'
Disturbed sleep pattern related to increased physical activity, fear, anxiety, unfamiliar environment	Client maintains normal sleep pattern	Assess for sleep pattern disturbance (e.g. not feeling well rested, or interrupted sleep, irritability, yawning) Determine the client's usual sleep habits Discourage long naps during the day Provide diversional activities during the day time Instruct the client to avoid intake of foods and fluids high in caffeine (e.g. coffee, tea) in the evening

Contd...

Contd...

Nursing diagnosis	*Objective*	*Plan of action*
		Reduce environmental stimuli Provide a glass of warm milk before going to sleep Provide a dark, quiet, and comfortable atmosphere
Self-care deficit related to inability to take responsibility for meeting self-care needs, lack of awareness of personal needs, hyperactivity	Client performs self-care activities	Assess the deficits in self-care Develop a realistic plan for meeting self-care needs Assist with personal hygiene and appropriate dress and grooming Keep needed objects within easy reach Provide adequate time for doing self-care activities Provide positive reinforcement for proper dressing and grooming
Disturbed thought process related to biochemical imbalances	Client demonstrate decreased delusions. Client demonstrates decreased pressured speech, tangentiality, loosening of association.	Assess the disturbance in thought process Decrease the environmental stimuli Accept the patient as a person Do not focus into delusions Be sincere when communicating with the patient Don't argue with the patient or try to make him understand that delusions are not real Never convey to the patient that you accept the delusion as real Never make fun of the patient's beliefs Provide diversional activities Administer antipsychotics as prescribed
Disturbed sensory perception related to biochemical changes	Client demonstrates accurate perception of the environment	Observe client for hallucinatory behavior (laughing or talking to self) Accept the patient as he is Do not reinforce the hallucination. Use words such as 'the voices' instead of 'they' when referring to the hallucination Try to distract the client during hallucination Instruct the patient to listen to the radio or watch television Teach the patient to say loudly, 'Go away!' or 'Leave me alone' Reduce the environmental stimuli Do not reinforce the hallucination

Contd...

Contd...

Nursing diagnosis	*Objective*	*Plan of action*
		Provide diversional activities Maintain reality by focusing on real situations and people Administer antipsychotics as prescribed
Impaired social interaction related to biochemical changes, agitation, hyperactivity	Client maintains optimum social interaction	Assess the psychomotor activity. Provide a environment with low stimuli Recognize the manipulative behavior Set limits on impulsive behavior Ignore attempts by patient to argue Discuss the consequences of his behavior Provide solitary activities (writing, drawing) Give positive reinforcement for non-manipulative behavior

BIPOLAR MOOD (AFFECTIVE) DISORDERS

Bipolar mood disorders were earlier known as Manic Depressive Psychosis (MDP) (Fig. 10.1).

Refers to disorders in which there are two or more episodes in which mood and activity levels of patients are disturbed. This disturbance may be of an elevated mood, increased energy and activity (hypomania or mania) and sometimes lowering of mood, decreased energy and activity (depression).

Mood disorders are of two types- unipolar and bipolar disorders. In unipolar disorders, there are repeated episodes of depression, but in bipolar type, there are recurrent episodes of mania and depression.

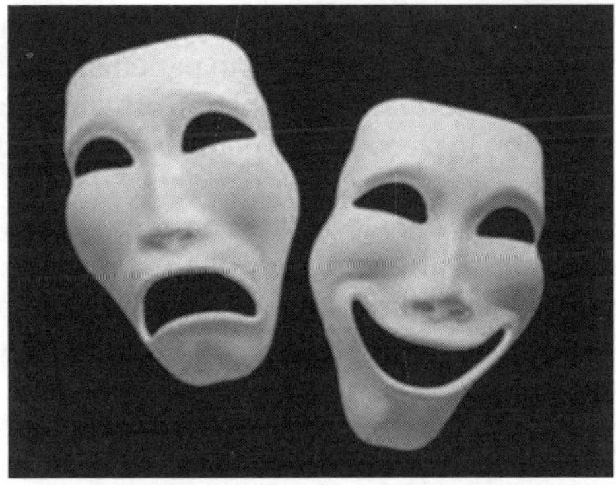

Fig. 10.1: Bipolar affective disorder

Classification of Bipolar Disorders

- **Bipolar I Disorder—**Characterized by mania in which symptoms are severe that needs immediate hospitalization. It will be followed by depressive episodes lasting at least 2 weeks.
- **Bipolar II Disorder—**The patient presents with depressive episodes and hypomanic episodes.

DEPRESSIVE EPISODE

In depressive episodes, the patient has low mood, reduced energy, and decrease in activity. Enjoyment, interest, and concentration are reduced.

Etiology of Depressive Episode

Etiology of mood disorders can be categorized into biological, psychological and social factors.

- **Biological theories:**
  - *Genetic hypothesis:* Genetic factors play an important role in the causation of mood disorders. If one parent is having depression, then the risk is 10–25% and if both parents are affected, the risk is doubled. A person whose first-degree relative has major depression the risk is 1.5 to 3% than the normal.
  - *Biochemical theories:* Dysfunction of certain neurotransmitters in the brain is postulated for the etiology of mood disorders. In depression, there is decrease in the amount of neurotransmitters like serotonin, norepinephrine and dopamine. In depression, there is reduced serotonin transmission. Low levels of a serotonin by product have been linked to a higher risk for suicide.
  - *Neurophysiological hypothesis:* Inhibitory functions of neurons may cause depression.
  - *Neuroendocrine hypothesis:* Dysfunction of hypothalamic—pituitary–adrenal axis is observed in patients with depression.
  - *Neuroanatomical changes:* Dysfunction of hypothalamus explains for the alteration in sleep and appetite in depressed clients.
- **Psychosocial theories:**
  - *Psychoanalytic theory:* Disturbances in mother-infant relationship during the first 10 to 18 months of life predispose to subsequent vulnerability to depression. Loss of libidinal object, intense craving for self-love has been postulated as the etiology for depression.
  - *Stress:* Stressful life events often act as a precipitating factor for the onset or relapse of mood disorders.
  - *Cognitive theories:* Aaron Beck has put forth the cognitive behavior theory which suggests that negative thoughts related

to self, others and the world (worthlessness, helplessness and hopelessness) causes depression.

Clinical Features

Depressive episode is characterized by:

- **Pervasive and persistent sadness:** Person feels sad throughout the day and it will be evident in all his activities. The depressed mood leads to decreased involvement in activities which were once pleasurable.
- **Decreased psychomotor activity:** Patients with depression presents with reduced thinking, decreased thought, speech and activity. Anxiety, irritability over minor events may be present.
- **Depressive cognitions:** Depressed mood is usually associated with negative thoughts related to self (worthlessness), others (helplessness) and future (hopelessness).
- **Physical symptoms:** Depressed person often presents with multiple physical complaints like heaviness of head, fatigue, dryness of mouth, constipation and body aches.
- **Biological functions:** Increase or decrease in appetite, weight and sleep is usually seen.
- **Psychotic features:** Delusions and hallucinations are seen in 15-20% of the patients with depression. Delusions of persecution, nihilistic, poverty and guilt are usually seen.
- **Suicide:** Suicidal risk is present in almost all depressed clients.

Management

- **Psychopharmacology**
  - *Antidepressants:* The commonly used antidepressants are tricyclic antidepressants (imipramine, amitriptyline and dothiepin) and selective serotonin reuptake inhibitors (fluoxetine and sertraline). When antidepressants are given, it will take 4–6 weeks to respond fully.
  - *Antipsychotics:* Antipsychotics like clozapine are used for the management of psychotic symptoms.
  - Lithium.
- **ECT:** This ECT is considered as the initial management of severe depression when it presents with suicidal ideation, not taking food or having catatonic/psychotic features.
- **Psychosocial therapies:** The psychosocial therapies effective in depression include:
  - Supportive psychotherapy
  - Interpersonal therapy
  - Behavior therapy

- Cognitive behavior therapy
- Marital therapy
- Family therapy.

Recurrent Depressive Disorder (RDD)

Characterized by repeated (at least two) depressive episodes.

PERSISTENT MOOD DISORDER

It is characterized by persistent mood symptoms that occurs for most of the day for at least 2 years (at least 1 year for children and adolescents).

Types of Persistent Mood Disorder

- **Cyclothymia:** It refers to persistent mood disorder in which multiple episodes of mild depression and elation occurs. Cyclothymia closely resembles bipolar mood disorder, but the symptoms are less severe and of long duration.
- **Dysthymia:** Dysthymic Disorder (dysthymia) is now replaced by the term *persistent depressive disorder (DSM 5).* Persistent depressive disorder is characterized by a depressed mood that occurs for most of the day. The symptoms of dysthymia are mild when compared to depressive disorder, but lasts for a longer duration. Dysthymia was also known as neurotic depression and depressive neurosis.

Difference between neurotic and psychotic depression are shown in Table 10.4.

Table 10.4: Difference between neurotic and psychotic depression

Characteristics	*Neurotic depression*	*Psychotic depression*
Other names	Exogenous depression Neurotic depression Dysthymia	Endogenous depression
Causes	Environmental factors/ Stressful events	Genetic factors
Clinical features	Difficulty in initiating sleep Prefers to be in group Depressive symptoms worsens in the evening Psychotic symptoms (Hallucination and delusion) absent	Difficulty in maintaining sleep Prefers to be alone Symptoms uniform throughout the day Psychotic symptoms present
Treatment	Psychotherapy Antidepressants Anxiolytics	Antidepressants Antipsychotics ECT
Prognosis	Good	Poor

INVOLUTIONAL MELANCHOLIA

This is a type of severe depression seen during involutional period (40–65 years). Characteristic features include agitation, delusion of persecution, hallucination, anorexia, insomnia and fatigue. They may also present with nihilistic and hypochondriacal delusions.

Prognosis

The prognosis of mood disorders is better when compared to schizophrenia. Good prognostic factors include well-adjusted premorbid personality, severe depression, acute onset and good response to treatment (Table 10.5).

Nursing Management

Table 10.5: Nursing care plan for a client with depression

Nursing diagnosis	*Objective*	*Intervention*
Risk for self-directed injury related to suicidal ideations, depressive thoughts	Client remains free from self-directed injury.	Observe client's behavior frequently. Observe for suicidal behaviors: Verbal statements, such as 'I am' going to kill myself' or nonverbal behaviors such as giving away valuable items Determine suicidal intent and methods. Ask, 'Do you plan to kill yourself?' and 'How do you plan to do it?' Obtain verbal or written contract for no suicide Remove all dangerous objects from client's environment Maintain low level of stimuli in client's environment (low lighting, few people and low noise level) Keep the patient near the nurses' station Avoid giving dress which has long sleeves Ensure that the patient consume medication Keep medicines under safe custody Administer tranquilizing medications as prescribed
Imbalanced nutrition less than body requirements related to loss of appetite	Client maintains optimum nutritional status	Assess the dietary pattern Check the weight daily Provide foods that are easily chewed, fortified liquids Consider the likes and dislikes of the patient

Contd...

Contd...

Nursing diagnosis	*Objective*	*Intervention*
		Ensure that client receives small, frequent meals including a bedtime snack, rather than three larger meals Do not tell the client that he or she will get sick or die from not eating or drinking Stay with client during meals Give positive reinforcement when he takes food
Self-care deficit (bathing, toileting, dressing) related to perceptual or cognitive impairment, anxiety.	Client establishes adequate personal hygiene.	Assess for the self-care abilities Initiate dressing and grooming tasks in the morning Maintain a routine for dressing, grooming, and hygiene Be gentle but firm in setting limits regarding time spent in bed Set specific times when the client must be up in the morning Provide positive feedback on performing the tasks
Disturbed sleep pattern related to hopelessness, perceived or actual threat	Client attains normal sleeping pattern	Assess the sleeping patterns Discourage sleep during the day Provide diversional activities on a structured, daily schedule Provide warm baths, back rubs Teach and instruct to do relaxation exercises Restrict intake of caffeinated drinks, such as tea and coffee Administer sedative medications as prescribed Administer antidepressant as prescribed
Disturbed thought process related to biochemical imbalances	Client demonstrate decreased delusions.	Assess the disturbance in thought process Decrease the environmental stimuli Accept the patient as a person Do not focus into delusions Be sincere when communicating with the patient Do not argue with the patient or try to make him understand that delusions are not real

Contd...

Contd...

Nursing diagnosis	*Objective*	*Intervention*
		Never convey to the patient that you accept the delusion as real Never make fun of the patient's beliefs Provide diversional activities Administer antipsychotics as prescribed
Disturbed sensory perception related to biochemical changes	Client demonstrates accurate perception of the environment	Observe client for hallucinatory behavior (laughing or talking to self) Accept the patient as he is Do not reinforce the hallucination Use words such as 'the voices' instead of 'they' when referring to the hallucination Try to distract the client during hallucination Instruct the patient to listen to the radio or watch television Teach the patient to say loudly, 'Go away!' or 'Leave me alone' Reduce the environmental stimuli Do not reinforce the hallucination Provide diversional activities Maintain reality by focusing on real situations and people Administer antipsychotics as prescribed
Chronic low self-esteem related to lack of approval, unsatisfactory parent-child relationship, negative reinforcement	Client exhibit increased feelings of self-worth	Explore with the client his or her abilities and strengths Assist client in identifying positive aspects of self Encourage the client to become involved ward interactions and activities When the patient conveys negative thoughts repeatedly, ask the patient to talk about positive topic after the negative content Spend time with client Initially provide simple activities that can be accomplished easily Start with a solitary activity, progress to group recreational therapy sessions Give the client positive feedback for participation Give positive reinforcement for development of more adaptive coping behaviors

Contd...

Contd...

Nursing diagnosis	*Objective*	*Intervention*
Impaired social interaction related to low self-worth, inadequate social skills	Client initiates interactions with others.	Assess the social interaction of the patient Talk with the client about his or her interactions Initially, interact with the client on a one-to-one basis Introduce the client to other clients in the ward Teach and encourage the client about social skills such as approaching another client for an interaction, appropriate conversation topics, and active listening Provide positive reinforcement for initiating conversation
Ineffective individual coping related to crisis	Client adopts effective coping strategies	Assess the client's perception of current situation Assess previous methods of coping with life's problems Set limits on his behavior Encourage verbalization of feelings, fears and anxiety Explore alternative coping strategies Teach the client about positive coping strategies and stress management skills, such as physical exercise, expressing feelings verbally or in writing Provide positive feedback

CONCLUSION

Mood disorders include disorders which involve severe disturbance in mood. Nurses can render quality care to clients with mood disorders by proper assessment, psychoeducation, physical care and prevention of relapse.

BIBLIOGRAPHY

1. Ahuja N. A Short Textbook of Psychiatry (7th ed). New Delhi: Jaypee Brothers Medical Publishers (P) Ltd, 2011.
2. American Psychiatric Association. Diagnostic and Statistical Manual of Mental Disorders (5th ed). Washington DC, 2013.
3. Halter, Margaret J Varcarolis, Elizabeth M (Eds). Varcarolis' Foundations of Psychiatric Mental Health Nursing: A Clinical Approach. St Louis, Mo: Elsevier, 2014.

4. Kapoor B. Textbook of Psychiatric Nursing. Delhi: Kumar Publishing House, 2014.
5. Schultz MJ, Videbeck LS. Lippincott's Manual of Psychiatric Nursing Care Plans. Philadelphia: Wolters Kluwer, 2012.
6. Theodore DD. Textbook of Mental Health Nursing. India: Elsevier, 2015.
7. Townsend CM. Nursing Diagnoses in Psychiatric Nursing: Care Plans and Psychotropic Medications (8th ed.). Philadelphia: FA Davis company, 2011.
8. Vyas JN, Ghimire RS. Textbook of Postgraduate Psychiatry (3rd ed.). New Delhi: Jaypee Brothers Medical Publishers (P) Ltd, 2016.
9. World Health Organization. The ICD-10 Classification of Mental and Behavioral Disorders: Clinical Descriptions and Diagnostic Guidelines. Geneva: World Health Organization, 1992.

CHAPTER 11 Neurotic, Stress-related and Somatoform Disorders

DEFINITION

Neurosis is a term generally used to describe a nonpsychotic mental illness which triggers feelings of distress and anxiety and impairs functioning (Encyclopaedia of mental disorders). The word neurosis is not used by ICD-10 and DSM V classification. Differences between neurosis and psychosis are shown in Table 11.1.

Table 11.1: Difference between neurosis and psychosis

Psychosis	*Neurosis*
Definition Mental illness in which reality testing and adaptation to life is markedly impaired	A non-psychotic mental illness which triggers feelings of distress and anxiety and impairs functioning
Cause Caused by organic factors and psychological factors	Predominantly by stressful factors
Clinical features • Reality testing is affected • Disturbances in affect is present • Disorders of perception–hallucination and illusion present • Disorders of thought—delusions, flight of ideas are present • Judgment is impaired • Marked impairment in memory and concentration • Insight is absent	• Reality testing is not affected • Affect is not affected • Hallucination and illusion are absent • Disorders of thought are absent • Judgment is not affected • Not affected • Insight present
Treatment Antipsychotics Electroconvulsive therapy (ECT) Psychotherapy	Antidepressants, Anxiolytics Psychotherapy
Prognosis Poor	Good
Recurrence Chance is more	Chance is less

CLASSIFICATION

F40-48 Neurotic, stress-related, and somatoform disorders:
- F40—Phobic anxiety disorders
- F41—Other anxiety disorders
- F42—Obsessive-compulsive disorder
- F43—Reaction to severe stress, and adjustment disorders
- F44—Dissociative [conversion] disorders
- F45—Somatoform disorders
- F48—Other neurotic disorders.

PHOBIC ANXIETY DISORDERS

Phobia is defined as an irrational fear of a specific object, situation or activity often leading to avoidance of that object, situation or activity.

Types of Phobia

- **Agoraphobia:** In this type of phobia, person has fear of open places. This is the commonest type of phobia seen in clinical practice.
- **Social phobia:** Irrational fear of participating in activities or social interaction manifested as fear to eat in public or to public speaking.
- **Specific phobia:** Person has irrational fear of a specific object or situation. Examples of specific phobia are spiders (arachnophobia), insects (entomophobia), heights (acrophobia) and closed spaces (claustrophobia).

ANXIETY

Anxiety is a state of apprehension or unease arising out of anticipation of fear. Fear is an apprehension in response to an external danger, whereas in anxiety the danger is mostly unknown.

Anxiety disorders are one of the common psychiatric disorders. Anxiety disorders cause distress that often interferes with the ability to lead a normal life.

Levels of Anxiety

Levels of anxiety are shown in Table 11.2.

Table 11.2: Levels of anxiety

Symptoms	*Mild anxiety*	*Moderate anxiety*	*Severe anxiety*	*Panic anxiety*
Physiological symptoms	Tachycardia, hypertension, diarrhea, cold and clammy skin	Symptoms of mild anxiety are increased. Urinary urgency will also be present	Symptoms are severe. Dilated pupils and decreased perception to pain	Severity of symptoms is increased

Contd...

Contd...

Symptoms	*Mild Anxiety*	*Moderate anxiety*	*Severe anxiety*	*Panic anxiety*
Attention and concentration	Increased attention, but not able to concentrate	Concentration is decreased	Decreased perception	Attention and concentration is very much affected
Activity	Increased	Restless	Trembling, pacing up and down	May scream
Appetite	Decreased	Decreased	Very much decreased	No appetite
Speech	Normal	Volume and tone is increased	Asks for help	Speech will not be clear
Muscle tone	Tightened	Tensed	Tense and rigid	Very poor

Types of Anxiety Disorders

- **Panic disorders (episodic paroxysmal anxiety):** This is characterized by recurrent episodes of acute anxiety. Symptoms usually occur unexpectedly and it is more common among females. Symptoms include palpitations, chest pain, choking and depersonalization.
- **Generalized anxiety disorder:** The essential characteristic feature of this disorder is anxiety lasting more than 6 months, which is generalized and persistent. Symptoms include feelings of nervousness, tremors, muscular tension, sweating, palpitations and dizziness.

Etiology

The etiology for phobic anxiety disorders can be categorized into:

- **Biological cause:** Rate of panic disorders among monozygotic twins is four times more when compared to dizygotic twins. Anxiety disorders are seen among 15–20% of the first degree relatives of patients with anxiety disorders.

  Inhibitory function of gamma-aminobutyric acid (GABA) is decreased in anxiety. Serotonin and dopamine are also involved in the causation of anxiety disorders.
- **Psychological factors:** According to behavior theory, anxiety and phobia are an unconditioned response to a painful stimulus.

  According to psychodynamic theory, a person uses defense mechanisms like repression, conversion, isolation and denial repeatedly to overcome anxiety. Use of displacement leads to phobia.
- **Sociocultural factors:** Stressful life events also play a major role in the causation of neurotic disorders. Anxiety is more common in high socioeconomic group.

Management

Anxiety disorders are managed with behavior therapy and anxiolytics like benzodiazepines (Alprazolam, Clonazepam). Antidepressants are also used.

OBSESSIVE-COMPULSIVE DISORDER

Definition

Obsessive-Compulsive Disorder (OCD) is a common, chronic and long-lasting disorder in which a person has uncontrollable, reoccurring thoughts (*obsessions*) and behaviors (*compulsions*) that he or she feels the urge to repeat over and over (National Institute of Mental Health).

Obsessions are thoughts, ideas or mental images that intrude repeatedly into one's mind causing anxiety.

Compulsions are repetitive and purposeful behaviors performed in response to obsessions (Table 11.3).

Table 11.3: Difference between obsession and compulsion

Obsession	*Compulsion*
An idea or image that intrudes repeatedly into mind	Repetitive and purposeful behaviors performed in response to obsessions
It is recognised as one's own idea	Behaviors are performed to prevent distress occurring out of obsession
Insight is present	Insight is present
Person tries to resist the thoughts, but often fails	Behavior is performed due to the strong desire to act

Etiology

The etiology for obsessive-compulsive disorder include:

- **Biological factors:** Imbalance in serotonin and glutamate is involved in the etiology of obsessive-compulsive disorder. OCD is seen in 5–7% of first degree relatives of OCD patients.
- **Psychological factors:** Behavior theory states that obsessions are conditioned stimuli to anxiety and compulsions are the learned behavior to reduce the anxiety associated with obsessions.

  According to psychodynamic theory, use of defense mechanisms like isolation, undoing and displacement produces obsessive-compulsive symptoms.
- **Sociocultural factors:** Environmental stressors may act as a precipitating factor for OCD. Obsessive-compulsive disorders are common in high socioeconomic group.

Vicious Cycle of OCD

OCD occurs in a vicious cycle as depicted below (Fig. 11.1)

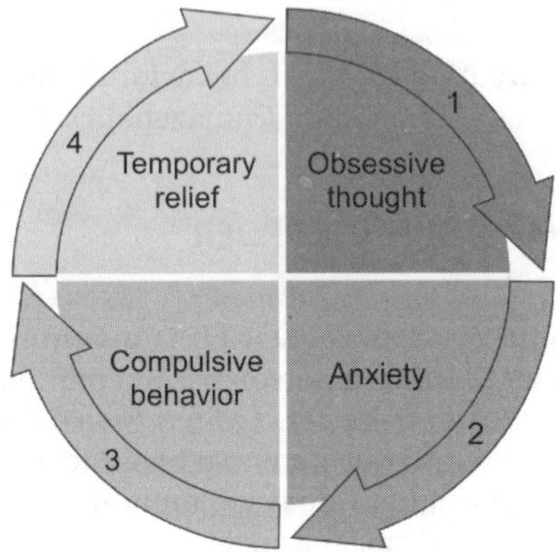

Fig. 11.1: The vicious cycle of OCD

Symptoms

Obsession

- Repeated unwanted ideas
- Fear of contamination
- Aggressive impulses
- Persistent sexual thoughts.

Compulsive Behaviors

- Constant checking
- Constant counting
- Cleaning of objects
- Repeatedly washing
- Constantly checking the stove or door locks
- Arranging things in a particular way.

Management

- **Psychotherapy:** This include behavior therapy—modeling and systematic desensitization. Exposure and response prevention is a type of behavior therapy used in OCD. Patients is exposed to objects and situation that produce anxiety. Gradually anxiety associated with these objects are reduced. In response prevention, patients with OCD are instructed not to do the ritual activity so as to reduce anxiety.
- **Psychopharmacology**: Anxiolytics, antidepressants and antipsychotics.
- **Electroconvulsive therapy (ECT)**: ECT is indicated if there is associated suicidal ideation or patient is not responding to other treatment modalities.

REACTION TO SEVERE STRESS AND ADJUSTMENT DISORDERS

Post-traumatic Stress Disorder (PTSD)

Post-traumatic stress disorder is characterized by recurrent and intrusive thoughts ('flashbacks'). Persons with PTSD exhibit emotional numbing such as feeling detached from others and have symptoms such as irritability, exaggerated startle response and insomnia. Usually tries to avoid situation that produce thoughts of the stressful event. Anxiety and depression are commonly associated.

Treatment of PTSD includes supportive psychotherapy, drugs such as antidepressants and anxiolytics.

Dissociative (Conversion) Disorders

The term hysteria was used previously, now it has been replaced as dissociative (conversion) disorder in ICD-10 classification and as conversion and dissociative disorders in DSM-5.

Dissociative disorders are characterized by disturbance in consciousness, memory and identity in which onset is usually sudden and recovery is abrupt. There is a precipitating stress before the onset.

Types of Dissociative Disorders (Table 11.4)

Table 11.4: Types of dissociative disorders

Types of dissociative disorders	*Features*
Dissociative identity disorder	Dissociative identity disorder was earlier known as multiple personality disorder. In dissociative identity disorder there is existence of two or more personality states that are different in behavior and thinking.
Dissociative amnesia	This is the commonest type of dissociative disorder. The main clinical feature is loss of memory, usually of important recent event. No underlying organic mental disorder. The amnesia is usually occurs after traumatic events, such as accidents and can last from minutes to days.
Depersonalization disorder	Depersonalization is a condition in which a person feels detached from oneself. The person feels that he as well as the external world is not real. Depersonalization is seen in depression, hypochondriasis and temporal lobe epilepsy.
Dissociative fugue	A disorder in which patient goes away from his home and adopts a new identity. During this time, the person has amnesia about the past life. Onset is sudden and usually follows a stressful event.

Conversion Disorder

Conversion disorder is a disorder characterized by the presence of one or more symptoms suggesting the presence of a neurological disorder that cannot be explained by any known neurological or medical disorders.

Onset is usually sudden and occurs following stressful event. Symptoms involve motor or sensory function. Detailed physical examination and investigations do not reveal any pathology. When conversion symptoms occur, the individual has both primary gain (avoidance of the fearful situation) and a secondary gain (attention and sympathy from others). Example—A lady living in a joint family suddenly develops paralysis of hands thus she has two gains—primary gain (escape from household responsibility) and a secondary gain (attention and sympathy from other members in the family).

Clinical Features

The clinical features can be categorized as sensory, motor and visceral symptoms.

- **Sensory symptoms:** Include anesthesia (loss of sensation), hypoesthesia (partial loss of sensitivity), hyperesthesia (excessive sensation) and paresthesia (sensation such as tingling).

  Glove anesthesia, deafness and blindness are also experienced. This disorder is called dissociative sensory disorders.
- **Motor symptoms:** Hysterical fit is one of the most common motor symptoms of conversion disorder. Hysterical fits is known as dissociative convulsions. Characteristic features of hysterical fits are that it can occur at any time and place, they do not bite their tongue, no loss of consciousness and injury will be very rare.

  Dissociative motor disorders are characterized by paralysis or abnormal movements. Hemiplegia, astasia-abasia (inability to stand or walk), tremors and tics are common symptoms of dissociative motor disorders.

Management

Management of dissociative disorders include:

- Behavior therapy
- Psychotherapy

This is the treatment of choice for dissociative disorders (e.g. free association, supportive psychotherapy, hypnosis).

Somatoform Disorders

Somatoform disorders are characterized by presence of physical symptoms which do not have any adequate physical basis and persistent request for investigations and treatment despite the assurance from physician.

Classification of Somatoform Disorders

- **Somatization disorder:** Characterized by the presence of multiple physical symptoms such as abdominal pain, nausea, vomiting and tingling. These symptoms are chronic, but there will be no underlying physical disorder.
- **Hypochondriacal disorder:** The disorder is characterized by a persistent preoccupation with the fear of developing one or more serious physical disorders. The fear is based on the fault interpretation of normal signs and sensations. Physical examination and investigation does not reveal any physical disorder, but the fear and convictions persist despite the reassurance.
- **Somatoform autonomic dysfunction:** These disorders present with symptoms of organ system that is controlled by autonomic nervous system (gastrointestinal, cardiovascular and respiratory system) in the absence of a physical disorder.

Treatment

- Supportive psychotherapy
- Behavior therapy
- Drug therapy—Anxiolytics and antidepressants if underlying anxiety and depression is present.

Other Neurotic Disorders

- **Neurasthenia:** The person with neurasthenia presents with increased fatigue after minimum effort. Body weakness, multiple aches, tension headaches, irritability and dyspepsia are usually reported.
- **Depersonalization-derealization syndrome:** Depersonalization refers to the alteration in the perception of self, so that feeling of one's reality is lost. Derealization refers to the alteration in the perception of environment, so that the feeling of one's own environment is lost (Table 11.6).

Psychosomatic Disorders

Psychosomatic means mind (psyche) and body (soma). The term psychosomatic was first used by Johann Christian Heinroth. Psychophysiological disorders were renamed as psychosomatic disorders in DSM-II. In ICD-10, it is included under somatoform disorders.

Definition

Psychosomatic disorders are a group of diseases characterized by physical symptoms that are caused by emotional factors and involve a single organ system, usually under autonomic nervous system control. The systems affected are respiratory, gastrointestinal, cardiovascular, neurological, genitourinary, musculoskeletal, endocrine and integumentary system.

Etiology

Predisposing Factors

Change in the neuroanatomy, neurotransmitter imbalances and altered brain function has a major role in the causation of psychosomatic disorders.

Precipitating Factors

These factors include conflicts, stress, loss and bereavement.

Types of Psychosomatic Disorders (Table 11.5)

Table 11.5: Psychosomatic disorders involving different organ system

Organ system involved	*Psychosomatic disorders*
Gastrointestinal system	Peptic ulcer, irritable bowel syndrome, ulcerative colitis, obesity
Cardiovascular system	CAD, hypertension, myocardial infarction
Respiratory system	Hyperventilation, asthma
Musculoskeletal system	Rheumatoid arthritis, low backache
Nervous system	Headaches, migraine
Integumentary system	Neurodermatitis, psoriasis, pruritis
Genitourinary system	Dysmenorrhea, amenorrhea, prostatitis, urethritis
Endocrine system	Diabetes mellitus, hyperthyroidism

Management

Medical treatment is to be initiated for the disease. Psychotherapy, family therapy, behavior therapy and relaxation training are effective.

Nursing Management

Table 11.6: Nursing care plan of a client with neurotic disorders

Nursing diagnosis	*Objective*	*Nursing intervention*
Anxiety related to actual or perceived threat	Client remains free from anxiety	Assess the level of anxiety. Maintain a calm, non-threatening manner. Establish a trusting nurse-patient relation. Stay with the client at times of anxiety. Shift the client to a quiet room with less stimuli. Reassure the client. Assume a calm manner. Teach and encourage the client to perform relaxation exercises such as deep breathing, progressive muscle relaxation and guided imagery. Administer medications as prescribed.

Contd...

Contd...

Nursing diagnosis	*Objective*	*Nursing intervention*
Fear related to threatening stimuli	Client performs in presence of phobic object or situation	Assess the fear of the client. Discuss the client's perception of threatening stimuli. Encourage client to identify feelings contributing to irrational fears. Instruct the client to substitute negative thoughts with positive ones. Ask the client to stop, wait, and not to escape from feared situation as soon as experienced. Encourage the use of relaxation exercises. Administer anxiolytics as prescribed.
Imbalanced nutrition less than body requirements related to loss of appetite	Client maintains optimum nutritional status	Assess the dietary pattern. Check the weight daily. Provide foods that are easily chewed, fortified liquids. Consider the likes and dislikes of the patient. Ensure that client receives small, frequent meals, including a bedtime snack, rather than three larger meals. Stay with client during meals. Give positive reinforcement when he takes food.
Disturbed sleep pattern related to hopelessness.	Client attains normal sleeping pattern	Assess the sleeping patterns. Discourage sleep during the day. Provide diversional activities on a structured, daily schedule. Provide warm baths, back rubs. Teach and instruct to do relaxation exercises. Restrict intake of caffeinated drinks, such as tea and coffee. Administer sedative medications as prescribed. Administer antidepressant as prescribed.
Self-care deficit related to excessive ritualistic behavior, irrational fear	Client performs self-care activities	Instruct client to perform normal activities of daily living (ADLs) to his or her level of ability. Encourage independence, but assist when client is unable to perform. Offer recognition and positive reinforcement for independent behavior. Show client how to perform activities with when there is difficulty.

Contd...

Contd...

Nursing diagnosis	*Objective*	*Nursing intervention*
Ineffective coping related to maturational crisis.	Client adopts effective coping strategies	Assess the anxiety of the client. First meet the client's dependency needs as necessary. Encourage independence. Provide positive reinforcement for independent behaviors. Gradually reduce the amount of time allotted for ritualistic behavior. Do not criticize or blame the patient when he does ritualistic behavior. Provide positive reinforcement when he performs non-ritualistic behavior.

CONCLUSION

Nurse should establish a trusty relation with patients with neurotic disorders so that they will express their feelings freely. Positive feedback is to be given to those clients when they adopt healthy coping strategies.

BIBLIOGRAPHY

1. Ahuja N. A Short Textbook of Psychiatry (Seventh edition). New Delhi: Jaypee Brothers Medical Publishers (P) Ltd, 2011.
2. American Psychiatric Association. Diagnostic and Statistical Manual of Mental Disorders (5th ed). Washington DC.
3. Neurosis - Encyclopedia of Mental Disorders http://www.minddisorders.com/Kau-Nu/Neurosis.html
4. Halter, Margaret J Varcarolis, Elizabeth M (Eds). Varcarolis' Foundations of Psychiatric Mental Health Nursing: A Clinical Approach. St. Louis, MO: Elsevier, 2014.
5. Kapoor B. Textbook of Psychiatric Nursing. Delhi: Kumar Publishing House, 2014.
6. Schultz MJ, Videbeck LS. Lippincott's Manual of Psychiatric Nursing Care Plans. Philadelphia: Wolters Kluwer, 2012.
7. Theodore DD. Textbook of Mental Health Nursing. India: Elsevier, 2015.
8. Townsend CM. Nursing Diagnoses in Psychiatric Nursing Care Plans and Psychotropic Medications (8th edition). Philadelphia: FA Davis Company, 2011.
9. Vyas JN, Ghimire RS. Textbook of Postgraduate Psychiatry (Third edition). New Delhi: Jaypee Brothers Medical Publishers (P) Ltd, 2016.
10. World Health Organization. The ICD-10 Classification of Mental and Behavioral Disorders: Clinical Descriptions and Diagnostic Guidelines. Geneva: World Health Organization, 1992.

CHAPTER 12

Personality Disorders

INTRODUCTION

Personality of an individual can be viewed in many aspects as—one's values, interests, attitudes and beliefs, behavior and sometimes as physical appearance also. But personality is the sum total of one's behavior, which is the combination of inherited and acquired characteristics that make a person unique.

Personality is the relatively stable or permanent pattern of behavior that include one's thoughts, perception, and interactions, which make one different from others.

PERSONALITY DISORDER

Personality becomes disordered when the behavior pattern becomes exaggerated and maladaptive. They will have difficulty to establish and maintain intimate relationship due to poor social skills. A few people with personality disorder suffer from painful feelings, but some of them are able to maintain relationships and career.

Definition

Personality disorders are deeply ingrained maladaptive behavior pattern characterized by difficulty to form enduring personal relationships and social functioning, that begin in the teenage years or young adulthood.

Epidemiology

Prevalence of personality disorder in India is 0–2.8% (Reddy and Chandrasekhar, 1998). It is more in males, but these problems are usually under reported.

Etiology

The exact etiology of personality disorder is unknown. But a combination of biological, psychological and social or environmental factors contributes to it.

Biological Causes

Genetic Factors

Twin and adoptive studies show the genetic predisposition for antisocial personality disorder. Monozygotic twins are more prone to develop personality disorders than dizygotic twins. If a biologically predisposed person have some crisis, it may trigger personality disorder.

Neurobiology—rapidly increasing changes in brain structure and functions are related to psychotic symptoms in schizotypal personality disorder.

Psychological Factors

Psychodynamic theories: As per these theories, the deficiencies in ego and superego development are the base of personality disorder. This deficiency may be due to problems in mother child relationships (overprotection or neglect from mother or early separation from mother).

Social/Environmental Factors

Family, environment, physical or sexual abuse are some of these factors. Abuse in childhood adds the risk of borderline personality disorder.

CLASSIFICATION OF PERSONALITY DISORDERS

ICD-10 Classification of Personality Disorders (F60–F69)

F60 – Specific personality disorders
F60.0 – Paranoid personality disorder
F60.1 – Schizoid personality disorder
F60.2 – Dissocial personality disorder
F60.3 – Emotionally unstable personality disorder
F60.30 – Impulsive type
F60.31 – Borderline type
F60.4 – Histrionic personality disorder
F60.5 – Anankastic personality disorder (obsessive compulsive)
F60.6 – Anxious avoidant personality disorder
F60.7 – Dependent personality disorder
F60.8 – Other specific personality disorders
F60.9 – Personality disorder, unspecified

These conditions are not due to brain damage or disease or psychiatric disorder, but have some general criteria.

General Criteria

- Abnormal behavior pattern is long lasting—not episodic like mental illness.

- Disharmonious attitude and behavior that involve affectivity, impulse-control, ways of thinking, perception and relationships.
- Abnormal behavior pattern is pervasive and maladaptive to affect personal and social situations.
- Manifestations occur in childhood or adolescence and persist in adulthood.
- Disorder causes personal distress in later stages.
- Disorder may be associated with problems in social and occupational functioning.

F60.0: PARANOID PERSONALITY DISORDER

Typical feature is suspiciousness and pervasive distrust to others. Prevalence of this is 0.5–2.5% of general population.

Features

- Pervasive distrust with suspiciousness.
- Sensitive and argumentative.
- Without justification, they show suspicion to spouse or friends.
- They appear guarded, tense and may avoid involvement in groups. They scan the environment and for clues of betrayal or attack.
- Tendency to bear grudges persistently and refuses to forgive insults.
- Ideas of reference.
- Tendency to experience self-importance.
- Tendency to distort experiences or neutral actions of others.

Prognosis

This personality disorder tends to be lifelong. In some people, it leads to paranoid schizophrenia. They will have problems in adjusting with others in work and in family life.

Treatment

Psychotherapy will be useful. Pharmacotherapy is useful in managing anxiety and agitation. Severe agitation and delusional thinking can be treated with antipsychotics.

F60.1: SCHIZOID PERSONALITY DISORDER

Characteristic feature is social withdrawal or detachment from others.

Other Features

- Restricted emotional expressions/emotionally cold.
- Detachment from others and inability to enjoy close relations. They keep distance from their family members also.

- Interest in solitary activities.
- Lack of interest in sexual experiences.
- Indifferent to praise or criticism and is unable to experience pleasure.
- They are self-absorbed or aloof.

Prevalence

Though the prevalence of this is not clear, it affects 7.5% of general population.

Schizoid personality disorder also starts in early childhood and is long lasting, but may not be lifelong.

Management—there is no specific drug. Psychotherapy—individual/group/family therapy is useful.

SCHIZOTYPAL PERSONALITY DISORDER

This is characterized by odd or magical thinking, eccentric behavior and pervasive problems in social relations.

Other Features

Social anxiety, inability to make close relations, odd behavior/speech/ideas that influence behavior, inappropriate affect, suspiciousness, idea of reference, unusual perceptual experience, that are not consistent with cultural norms. They are not aware of own feelings, but aware and sensitive to other's feelings like anger. They are socially isolated.

Schizotypal can be considered as the premorbid personality of schizophrenia patients, some of them maintain it as stable personality.

Management

These people seek treatment once they become psychotic or depressed. This can be treated with small dose of antipsychotics.

Cognitive behavior therapy will be useful, if the individual is co-operative.

F60.2: DISSOCIAL PERSONALITY DISORDER (ANTISOCIAL)

It is also known as sociopath or psychopath and is characterized by long lasting antisocial behavior that violates social norms and other's rights and thus engages in criminal activities.

Features

- Violation of social norms
- Exploiting others by violating their rights
- Lack of empathy or lack of concern for others
- Irresponsible at school and work

- Irritable and aggressive behavior
- Impulsive behavior
- Lack of remorse/guilt
- Poor frustration tolerance
- Failure to learn from experience
- Inability to maintain a stable personal and sexual relationship.

In the beginning of childhood itself there will be history of lying, stealing, truancy, running away from home, fights, substance abuse and illegal activities (features of conduct disorder).

Promiscuity, spouse abuse, child abuse and substance abuse are some of the problems in adulthood.

Prevalence

It is most common among younger adults, mainly of urban areas. Prevalence is 3% in men and 1% in women. It is five times more common in first degree relatives of men with this disorder.

Management

It runs in unremitting course, but studies show that the disorder diminishes with age. Hospitalization for psychotherapy will be helpful. Self-help groups and therapeutic community settings, with environmental manipulation will be more useful.

Drug therapy must be done with special attention to prevent abuse.

F60.31: BORDERLINE PERSONALITY DISORDER

Lack of stability in interpersonal relations, self-image and affect with impulsivity that begins in early adulthood are the characteristic features.

Other Features

- Argumentative or sometime depressed.
- Intense and unstable emotions or mood.
- They feel both dependent and hostile.
- They view people as either nurturing type or hateful and sadistic type.
- Frequently shifts attachment from one person or group to another.
- Absence of sustaining, caring relationships.
- Dependent on those who are close and anger towards them when get frustrated.
- Impulsive behavior—self-injury, substance abuse, risky sexual relations, binge eating.
- Unpredictable behavior.

Prevalence of borderline personality disorder is 1–2% of general population.

Management

It is stable and patients do not change over time. These people show high incidence of major depression.

Behavior therapy to control impulses and anger outburst and to decrease the sensitivity to criticism. Individual psychotherapy and group therapy are also effective.

Antipsychotics are useful in anger, hostility and brief psychotic episode. Antidepressants are also used because these people are more prone to develop depression.

F60.4: HISTRIONIC PERSONALITY DISORDER

Long lasting attention seeking and self-dramatizing behavior is the characteristic of it. They maintain self-centered approach in personal relationships.

Features

- Attention and approval seeking behavior.
- Dramatic behavior.
- Exaggerated emotional response.
- Excessive sensitivity and disapproval to criticism.
- Over-concern with physical appearance.
- Craving for novelty and excitement.
- Seductive and will be the center of attention.
- Low frustration tolerance.
- Self-centered, lack of concern for others.
- Highly fluctuating emotional states.
- Easily influenced by others and falsely believe that relationships are intimate.

Prevalence is 2–3% in general population. It is more frequently diagnosed in women than in men, especially in separated or divorced.

Management

- As the age advances the symptoms become lesser.
- Psychotherapy—individual or group therapy will be effective.
- Pharmacotherapy as anxiolytics for anxiety and antidepresants for depression.

NARCISSISTIC PERSONALITY DISORDER

Characteristic features are pervasive pattern of grandiosity, desire for admiration, lack of empathy. It is seen from early adulthood.

Features

- Grandiosity/feeling of self-importance.
- Self-centered, sense of self-worth, and expect special attention or treatment.
- Disregard and lack of acceptance of others.
- Lack of empathy and arrogant nature.
- Sensitive to criticism.
- Make conflictual relationships that are superficial and exploits others.
- Ambitious for fame and daydreams about success and power.

Prevalence of it is 2–16% in the clinical population and less than 1% in the general population. These person's children have more risk for developing it.

Management

- It is chronic and difficult to treat.
- Psychotherapy with psychoanalytic approach will be helpful.
- These people are more prone for depression, and antidepressants will be useful.
- Lithium can be used in case of mood swings.

F60.5: OBSESSIVE-COMPULSIVE PERSONALITY DISORDER (ANANKASTIC PERSONALITY DISORDER)

Characteristic features are extreme orderliness, perfectionism and interpersonal control rather than openness, flexibility and efficiency.

Features

- Preoccupation with rules and regulations, orderliness, neatness, and perfectionism.
- Extreme conscientiousness leads to rigidity and inflexibility.
- Perfectionism delays task completion.
- Hard workers with less leisure activities and relationships.
- They rarely make mistakes and believe that their way is the right one.
- Put pressure on others to follow right moral principles, rigidity and stubbornness.
- Takes excess caution with feeling of excess doubts.

Prevalence

Males have higher rate as 5 times higher than females. More prevalent in highly educated, married and employed people. Usually associated with anxiety disorders.

Management

Course of it is unpredictable and variable. Depressive disorders of late onset may occur.

These people are often aware of their problem and seek treatment on their own.

Responds well to psychoanalytic psychotherapy, group therapy. Behavior therapy are also useful.

F60.6: ANXIOUS AVOIDANT PERSONALITY DISORDER

Characteristic features are extreme social anxiety with inadequate feeling that leads to social withdrawal.

Features

- Poor self-confidence and feeling of inferiority.
- Hypersensitivity to other's opinion—fear of criticism or rejection.
- Persistent tension and apprehension.
- Social anxiety and social withdrawal.

People with this disorder may have some psychiatric disorders like anxiety disorder, social phobia, obsessive-compulsive disorder, somatoform disorders and schizophrenia.

Management

With continuous and compassionate treatment, prognosis is good.

Long-term psychotherapy is needed because these people distrust others. Therapist has to empathize with the individual and must help him/her to identify the role of inferiority and inadequacy feeling and it is in connection with social anxiety and social withdrawal.

Cognitive behavior therapy will help in changing the distorted thought pattern. Group therapy also will be useful, as the person shows some improvement in interaction with others.

F60.7: DEPENDENT PERSONALITY DISORDER

Characteristic features are excessive need of care from others and it leads to submissive and clinging behavior and fear of separation that starts in early adulthood.

Features

- Low self-esteem, doubts about own capabilities leads to avoidance of positions of responsibilities.
- Anxious to assume leader's role.

- Always agree those whom they depend and tend to be submissive, passive and self-sacrificing.
- Helpless feeling and fear with break in the dependent relationship.

They need to find another person for nurturance and direction, or even prefer abusive relationships rather than being their own.

Management

These people have impaired social and occupational functioning due to the need for supervision, that arise from lack of self-confidence.

If they lose their dependent relationship, they may develop major depression, but prognosis is good with treatment.

Insight oriented therapies help the individual to recognize their strengths or abilities. With the support from the therapist, person become independent and self-reliant.

As these people are more prone to suffer from anxiety or depression, anxiolytics and antidepressants will be helpful in managing their symptoms.

DSM-5: CLASSIFICATION OF PERSONALITY DISORDER

According to DSM-5, there are 10 personality disorders that are grouped under Cluster A, Cluster B and Cluster C.

Cluster A: Odd or Eccentric

- Paranoid personality disorder
- Schizoid personality disorder
- Schizotypal personality disorder.

Cluster B: Dramatic, Emotional, or Erratic

- Antisocial personality disorder
- Borderline personality disorder
- Histrionic personality disorder
- Narcissistic personality disorder.

Cluster C: Anxious or Fearful

- Avoidant personality disorder
- Dependent personality disorder
- Obsessive-compulsive personality disorder.

NURSING CONSIDERATIONS IN PERSONALITY DISORDERS

Most of these persons are coming to hospital with the problems like anxiety, depression, adjust problems or family problems.

Persons with personality disorder need special attention and empathy. Most of these persons have distrust towards others and poor social interaction. So dealing with these persons will be a difficult task for the nurse.

- Nurse should establish a trusting relationship by empathizing with them through active listening, observations and identification of their personal feelings.
- Convey an accepting attitude and approach, while dealing with the patient.
- Explain the routine and rules in the hospital settings, and maintain consistency in all dealings.
- Provide a safe environment because impulsivity in these patients may lead to self-mutilating behavior. Remove all hazardous objects from the environment. Set limits in behavior whenever needed.
- Supervise and direct in self-care, if essential.
- Identify the inappropriate behavior and discuss about it in terms of suggestions for alternative behavior. Discuss how his/her behavior affects others and help him to seek adaptive behavior.
- Maintain a matter of fact approach in care. Do not neglect or over concern the patient.
- Talk with the patients an encourage to ventilate their feelings and thoughts.
- Find out the factors that cause acting out behavior or aggression. Passively observe for any signs of aggression—facial expressions, grinding the teeth, clenching of fist, loud speech, shouting, use of abusive words and destructive activities and intervene before escalation of behavior.
- Watch for manipulative behavior and set limits by involving other team members also.
- Be honest in all dealings with the patient. Avoid whispering and unclear discussions in front of patient. Talk with clear, simple language.
- Give positive reinforcement then and there, for any positive change in behavior.
- Involve the patient in the unit activities.
- Observe for suicidal ideations/behavior and manage accordingly.
- Advise the patient to keep a diary to note down the daily activities and any problem behavior, and it's consequences. This will help in gaining insight.
  Educate/train on management and prevention of such problem.
- Educate and assist the patient in problem-solving and better coping strategies.

- Assist in behavior modifications and other therapies.
- Provide a planned routine, include exercise, group activities, recreation and other activities of interest in the schedule.
- Administer medications and monitor for desired effects and side effects.
- Educate the family members regarding these patient's features and special concerns in dealings.

CONCLUSION

People with personality disorders present some problem—behaviors, that are inappropriate, and sometimes causes distress to self or others. Early identification and modification of these behaviors, through a team approach will be ideal, so that the individual will become a good citizen with self-worth and trust.

BIBLIOGRAPHY

1. Ahuja N. A Short Textbook of Psychiatry (Seventh edition). New Delhi: Jaypee Brothers Medical Publishers (P) Ltd, 2011.
2. American Psychiatric Association. Diagnostic and Statistical Manual of Mental Disorders (Fifth ed). Washington, DC, 2013.
3. Sreevani R. A Guide to Mental Health and Psychiatric Nursing (Third Edition). New Delhi: Jaypee Brothers Medical Publishers (P) Ltd, 2016.
4. Theodore DD. Textbook of Mental Health Nursing. India: Elsevier, 2015.
5. Townsend CM. Psychiatric Mental Health Nursing: Concepts of Care in Evidence-Based Practice (7th Edition). Philadelphia: FA Davis Company, 2012.
6. Vyas JN, Ghimire RS. Textbook of Postgraduate Psychiatry (Third edition). New Delhi: Jaypee Brothers Medical Publishers (P) Ltd, 2016.
7. World Health Organization. The ICD-10 Classification of Mental and Behavioral Disorders: Clinical Descriptions and Diagnostic Guidelines. Geneva: World Health Organization, 1992.

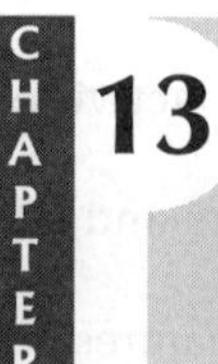

CHAPTER 13 Eating, Sleep and Sexual Disorders

F50-F59: BEHAVIORAL SYNDROMES ASSOCIATED WITH PHYSIOLOGICAL DISTURBANCES AND PHYSICAL FACTORS

F50	Eating disorders
F51	Non-organic sleep disorders
F52	Sexual dysfunction, not caused by organic disorder
F53	Mental and behavioral disorders associated with puerperium
F54	Psychological and behavioral factors associated with disorders or diseases
F55	Abuse of non-dependence-producing substances
F59	Unspecified

F50 EATING DISORDERS

A broad group of psychological disorders with abnormal eating behaviors leading to physiological effects from overeating or insufficient food intake.

Classification of Eating Disorders

F50.0	Anorexia nervosa
F50.2	Bulimia nervosa
F50.4	Overeating associated with other psychological disturbances
F50.5	Vomiting associated with other psychological disturbances
F50.8	Other eating disorders
F50.9	Eating disorder, unspecified

Anorexia Nervosa

Anorexia nervosa is a syndrome characterized by fear of gaining weight and significant body image disturbance.

Etiology

Biological Causes

First-degree female relatives and monozygotic twin offspring of patients with anorexia nervosa have higher rates of anorexia nervosa and bulimia nervosa. Children of patients with anorexia nervosa have a tenfold lifetime risk for anorexia nervosa than that of the general population.

Psychological Causes

Low self-esteem, disturbance of body image are important factors contributing to anorexia nervosa.

Social Causes

Influences of mass media, peer pressure are some of the social factors implicated in the etiology of anorexia nervosa.

Clinical Features

- Weight loss (body weight of at least 15% below the normal or expected weight for age and height).
- A self-perception of being too fat, with an intense fear of fatness.
- Body image disturbance
- Amenorrhea
- Thin hair
- Brittle nails
- Constipation
- Dry skin
- Dehydration

Complications

- Malnutrition
- Hypoalbuminemia
- Chronic inflammatory bowel disease
- Esophageal erosion
- Increased risk for infection

Treatment

Pharmacotherapy

- Antidepressants
- Antipsychotics

Psychotherapy

- Cognitive-behavior therapy
- Behavior therapy
- Family therapy

Bulimia Nervosa

Bulimia nervosa is characterized by recurrent episodes of binge eating followed by compensatory behaviors. Binge eating refers to eating much more quickly than usual, eating until uncomfortably full or eating a lot when not physically hungry. Compensatory measures include self-induced vomiting, use of diuretics or laxatives and dieting.

Clinical Features

- Recurrent episodes of overeating in which large amounts of food are consumed in short periods of time.
- Persistent preoccupation with eating and a strong desire or a sense of compulsion to eat (craving).
- Compensatory behavior to reduce weight (self-induced vomiting, alternating periods of starvation, use of drugs such as appetite suppressants)
- Weight loss
- Menstrual abnormalities or amenorrhea
- Fluid and electrolyte abnormalities
- Intermittent edema
- Erosion of the dental enamel.

Treatment

Pharmacotherapy

- Antidepressants

Psychotherapy

- Cognitive-behavior therapy
- Family therapy.

Nursing Management

- Imbalanced nutrition less than body requirements related to poor food intake, self-induced vomiting.
- Deficient fluid volume related to the self-induced vomiting or use of laxatives.
- Ineffective denial related to retarded ego development.
- Disturbed body image related to retarded ego development.
- Low self-esteem related to retarded ego development and dysfunctional family system.

Nursing Interventions

- Assess the dietary pattern
- Check the weight daily

- Maintain intake/output (I/O) chart
- Encourage to ventilate feelings and fear regarding the behavior
- Administer intravenous fluids
- Provide Ryle's tube feeding
- Provide balanced diet
- Encourage to adopt effective coping strategies
- Administer medications as prescribed.

F51: NON-ORGANIC SLEEP DISORDERS

Definition

Sleep disorder are abnormalities in the amount, quality, or timing of sleep and abnormal behavioral and physiological events occurring in association with sleep, specific sleep stages, or sleep-wake transitions.

Classification

F51.0	Non-organic insomnia
F51.1	Non-organic hypersomnia
F51.2	Non-organic disorder of the sleep-wake schedule
F51.3	Sleepwalking (somnambulism)
F51.4	Sleep terrors (night terrors)
F51.5	Nightmares
F51.8	Other non-organic sleep disorders
F51.9	Non-organic sleep disorder, unspecified.

International classification of sleep disorders (ICSD) classified sleep disorders into:

- Dyssomnia
- Parasomnia

I. DYSSOMNIA

A disorder in which there is disturbance in the amount, quality, or timing of sleep.

Types of Dyssomnia

1. Insomnia

Insomnia is defined as repeated difficulty with the initiation and maintenance, or quality of sleep.

Epidemiology

Ranging from 30–35%.

Causes of Insomnia

- **Use of psychoactive drugs** (such as stimulants)
- **Pain**
- **Life events** such as fear, stress, anxiety, emotional or mental tension, work problems, financial stress, birth of a child and bereavement.
- **Mental disorders** such as bipolar disorder, clinical depression, generalized anxiety disorder, post-traumatic stress disorder, schizophrenia, obsessive-compulsive disorder, dementia or alcoholism.
- **Medical conditions** such as hyperthyroidism and rheumatoid arthritis.
- **Poor sleep hygiene**, e.g. noise
- **Physical exercise**.

Treatment

- Medications
  - Anxiolytics
- Non-medical treatment and behavioral therapy
  - *Relaxation technique:* Relaxation therapy involves measures such as meditation, self-hypnosis, muscle relaxation or dimming the lights and playing soothing music prior to going to bed.
  - Yoga
  - *Sleep Hygiene:* The steps include:
    - Sleep as much as needed to feel rested.
    - Keep a regular sleep and awakening schedule.
    - Avoid naps
    - Exercise regularly at least 20 minutes daily, but not within 3 hours of bed time.
    - Do not drink caffeinated beverages in the night (tea, coffee, soft drinks, etc.)
    - Abstain from alcohol.
    - Avoid nicotine before bedtime and during the night.
    - Do not go to bed hungry.
    - Use the bedroom for sleeping; avoid doing non-sleep activities (for studying, watching television, or socializing on the telephone).
    - Adjust the environment in the room (lights, temperature, noise, etc.)
    - Set a relaxing routine to prepare for sleep. Avoid frustrating or provoking activities before bedtime and try to resolve worries before going to bed.

2. Hypersomnia

Hypersomnia is characterized by recurrent episodes of excessive daytime sleepiness or prolonged night-time sleep. It is also known as DOES (Disorder of Excess Somnolence).

Symptoms of Hypersomnia

- Persons with hypersomnia take nap repeatedly during the day, often at inappropriate times such as at work, during a meal, or in conversation.
- They fall asleep easily and sleep through the night but often have difficulty awakening in the morning.
- The daytime naps usually provide no relief from symptoms.
- Concentration and memory will be reduced.

Treatment of Hypersomnia

Treatment is symptomatic in nature.

- Changes in behavior (e.g. avoiding night work and social activities that delay bed time) and diet may offer some relief.
- Patients should avoid alcohol and caffeine.

II. PARASOMNIA

Parasomnias are undesirable physical phenomena that occur predominantly during sleep.

Types of Parasomnia

- **Sleep terror or night terror:** A night terror is characterized by feelings of terror or dread during the first several hours after sleep onset.
- **Nightmares:** Nightmares are frightening dreams that lead to awakenings from sleep.
- **Somnambulism:** Sleepwalking or somnambulism is a state of altered consciousness in which phenomena of sleep and wakefulness are combined.
- **Sleep related enuresis or bedwetting:** Refers to involuntary urination during sleep.
- **Bruxism:** Bruxism ('gnashing of teeth') is an involuntary, forceful grinding of teeth during sleep.
- **Somniloquy:** Somniloquy or sleep-talking refers to talking aloud in one's sleep.

Nursing Management (Table 13.1)

Table 13.1: Nursing care plan of a client with sleep disorders

Nursing diagnosis	*Objective*	*Nursing interventions*
Disturbed sleep pattern related to (specific medical condition), use of or withdrawal from substances, anxiety or depression, circadian rhythm disruptions, familial patterns	• Client will be able to achieve adequate, uninterrupted sleep. • Client will report feeling rested and demonstrate a sensation of well-being.	• Discourage strenuous exercise within one hour of bed time • Control intake of caffeine containing substances within 4 hours of bed time • Provide a high carbohydrate snack before bed time • Reduce environmental stimuli • Instruct the client not to use alcoholic beverages • Discourage smoking and other tobacco products near sleep time • Discourage day time napping • Encourage activities that prepare one for sleep: soft music, relaxation exercise or warm bath
Risk of injury related to excessive sleeping, sleep terrors, or sleepwalking	Client remains free from injury	• Keep the side rails of the bed up • Keep the bed in a low position • Equip the bed with a bell that is activated when the bed is excited • Keep a night light on and arrange the furniture in the bedroom in a manner that promote safety • Administer drug therapy as prescribed.

F52: SEXUAL DYSFUNCTION, NOT CAUSED BY ORGANIC DISORDER OR DISEASE

Sexual dysfunction consists of an impairment or disturbance in any of the phases of the sexual response cycle.

Some of sexual dysfunctions include the following:

- **Hypoactive Sexual Desire Disorder:** This disorder is defined as a persistent or recurrent deficiency or absence of sexual fantasies and desire for sexual activity.
- **Sexual Aversion Disorder:** This disorder is characterized by a persistent or recurrent extreme aversion to, and avoidance of, all (or almost all) genital sexual contact with a sexual partner.

- **Male Erectile Disorder:** This disorder is characterized by a persistent or recurrent inability to attain, or to maintain an adequate erection until completion of the sexual activity.
- **Dyspareunia:** Dyspareunia is defined as recurrent or persistent genital pain associated with sexual intercourse, in either a man or a woman that is not caused by vaginismus lack of lubrication, other general medical condition, or the physiological effects of substance use.
- **Vaginismus:** Vaginismus is characterized by an involuntary constriction of the outer one-third of the vagina, which prevents penile insertion and intercourse.

Management

- Pharmacotherapy
  - Antipsychotics
  - Antidepressants
  - Antianxiety drugs
- Psychotherapy
  - Behavior therapy
  - Group therapy.

F65: DISORDERS OF SEXUAL PREFERENCE

These disorders are included in F60–69 in ICD classification.

Paraphilia is characterized by the presence of sexual arousal in response to non-human object, which are not a part of normal sexual arousal.

Classification

F65.0	Fetishism
F65.1	Fetishistic transvestism
F65.2	Exhibitionism
F65.3	Voyeurism
F65.4	Pedophilia
F65.5	Sadomasochism
F65.6	Multiple disorders of sexual preference
F65.8	Other disorders of sexual preference
F65.9	Disorder of sexual preference, unspecified.

Fetishism

Fetishism involves recurrent, intense, sexual urges or behaviors, or sexually arousing fantasies involving the use of nonliving objects. This includes shoes, gloves and stockings.

Fetishistic Transvestism

Sexual arousal ocurs by wearing clothes of the opposite sex.

Exhibitionism

Exhibitionism is characterized by recurrent, intense, sexual urges, behaviors of at least 6-month duration, involving the exposure of one's genitals to an unsuspecting stranger.

Frotteurism

Frotteurism is the recurrent preoccupation with intense sexual urges or behaviors of at least 6-month duration involving touching or rubbing against a non-consenting person.

Pedophilia

The essential feature is presence of recurrent sexual urges, behaviors of at least 6-month duration, involving sexual activity with a prepubescent child.

Sexual Masochism

The identifying feature of sexual masochism is the occurrence of sexual arousal on inflicting physical harm to sexual partner.

Sexual Sadism

The essential feature is occurrence of sexual arousal on inflicting physical harm to oneself.

Voyeurism

This disorder is identified by recurrent, intense, sexual urges, behaviors, or sexually arousing fantasies, of at least 6-month duration, involving the act of observing an unsuspecting person who is naked or engaging in sexual activity.

Nursing Management

Nursing Diagnosis

- Sexual dysfunction related to conflict in relationship or certain biological or psychological contributing factors to the disorder evidenced by loss of sexual desire or ability to perform.
- Ineffective sexuality patterns related to conflicts with sexual orientation or variant preferences, evidenced by expressed dissatisfaction with sexual behaviors.

Nursing Interventions for Sexual Dysfunctions

- Assess client's sexual history and previous level of satisfaction in sexual relationship.
- Assess client's perception of the problem.
- Help client determine time dimension associated with the onset of the problem and discuss what was happening in life situation at that time.
- Assess client's level of energy.
- Review medication regimen; observe for side effects.
- Provide information regarding sexuality and sexual functioning.
- Refer for additional counseling or sex therapy if required.

Nursing Interventions for Ineffective Sexuality Patterns

- Take sexual history, noting client's expression of areas of dissatisfaction with sexual pattern.
- Assess areas of stress in client's life and examine relationship with sexual partner.
- Note cultural, social, racial, and religious factors that may contribute to conflicts regarding variant sexual practices.
- Be accepting and nonjudgmental.
- Assist therapist in plan of behavior modification.

CONCLUSION

Disturbances in the eating, sleep and sexual functions are encountered in clients with various mental as well as medical disorders. Awareness regarding the management of these disturbances is vital when rendering care to these clients.

BIBLIOGRAPHY

1. Ahuja N. A Short Textbook of Psychiatry (Seventh edition). New Delhi: Jaypee Brothers Medical Publishers (P) Ltd, 2011.
2. American Psychiatric Association. Diagnostic and Statistical Manual of Mental Disorders (5th edition). Washington, DC, 2013.
3. Halter, Margaret J Varcarolis, Elizabeth M (Eds). Varcarolis' Foundations of Psychiatric Mental Health Nursing: A Clinical Approach. St Louis, Mo: Elsevier, 2014.
4. International Classification of Sleep Disorders - European Society of classification of sleep disoders Available from www.esst.org/adds/ICSD.pdf
5. Kapoor B. Textbook of Psychiatric Nursing. Delhi: Kumar Publishing House, 2014.

6. Lalitha K. Mental Health and Psychiatric Nursing. Delhi: CBS Publishers, 2009.
7. Rawlins PR, Williams RS and Beck KC. Mental Health Psychiatric Nursing: A Holistic Life Cycle Approach. St Louis: Mosby, 1998.
8. Schultz MJ, Videbeck LS. Lippincott's Manual of Psychiatric Nursing Care Plans. Philadelphia: Wolters Kluwer, 2012.
9. Shives RL. Basic Concepts of Psychiatric-Mental Health Nursing. Philadelphia: Lippincott Williams and Wilkins, 2008.
10. Sreevani R. A Guide to Mental Health and Psychiatric Nursing (Third Edition). New Delhi: Jaypee Brothers Medical Publishers (P) Ltd, 2016.
11. Theodore DD. Textbook of Mental Health Nursing. India: Elsevier, 2015.
12. Townsend CM. Nursing Diagnoses in Psychiatric Nursing Care Plans and Psychotropic Medications (8th edition). Philadelphia: FA Davis Company, 2011.
13. Vyas JN, Ghimire RS. Textbook of Postgraduate Psychiatry (Third edition). New Delhi: Jaypee Brothers Medical Publishers (P) Ltd, 2016.
14. World Health Organization. The ICD-10 Classification of Mental and Behavioral Disorders: Clinical Descriptions and Diagnostic Guidelines. Geneva: World Health Organization 1992.

CHAPTER 14

Child and Adolescent Psychiatric Disorders

INTRODUCTION

Childhood psychiatric disorders are not easily diagnosed due to the less cognitive and verbal skills in them, and due to lack of knowledge about it. Like adults, children and adolescents also experience certain mental health problems. Neuropsychiatric disorders in infancy, childhood and in adolescence may persist to adulthood. Early detection of problems helps to treat this in childhood itself. Behavior modification, cognitive behavior therapy, play therapy and family therapy can bring out good results in childhood, if they are identified early.

Many psychiatric problems in children are manifested as developmental delay, emotional symptoms, conduct problems and impairment in socialization and relationships.

The ICD-10 Classification of Childhood and Adolescent Disorders

According to ICD-10, common childhood and adolescent disorders are classified as follows:

- F70-F79: Mental retardation
- F80-F89: Disorders of psychological development
- F90-F98: Behavioral and emotional disorders with onset in childhood and adolescence.

F70-F79: MENTAL RETARDATION

Mental retardation is a neurodevelopmental disorder with marked impairment in intellectual and adaptive functioning, and an IQ of less than 70. Mental retardation (MR) is also known as intellectual disability (ID).

ICD-10 Classification of Mental Retardation

- F70 – Mild mental retardation
- F71 – Moderate mental retardation
- F72 – Severe mental retardation
- F73 – Profound mental retardation.

Definitions

In DSM V mental retardation is named as intellectual disability or intellectual developmental disorder is defined as follows:

- Intellectual disability is a disorder with onset during the developmental period that includes both intellectual and adaptive functioning deficits in conceptual, social and practical domains (APA 2013).
- Mental retardation is the significantly sub-average intelligence with intelligent quotient (IQ) less than 70, and impairment in adaptive functioning that arises in the developmental period (< 18 years).

Epidemiology

According to WHO the overall prevalence of MR in the global scenario is 1–3% in 2001, and in Kerala, it is 0–1% of all children up to 6 years.

Etiological Factors

Etiological/predisposing factors of mental retardation can be broadly classified as primary causes and secondary causes.

I. Primary Causes

- **Genetic factors**
  - Inborn errors of metabolism like phenylketonuria.
  - Chromosomal disorders, e.g. Down syndrome and Klinefelter's syndrome.
  - Single-gene abnormalities like tuberous sclerosis and Neurofibromatosis.
  - Cranial malformations like microcephaly.
- **Developmental factors**
  - Maternal problems in pregnancy:
    - Use of drugs or alcohol by mother.
    - Viral infections (rubella or cytomegalovirus).
    - Endocrine disorders like hypothyroidism and hypoparathyroidism.
    - Malnutrition in pregnancy leading to fetal malnutrition and low birth weight.
    - Late pregnancy/aged pregnancy.
    - Complications of pregnancy—toxemia, diabetes, anemia and placental dysfunctions.
  - Problems during intranatal and postnatal factors can affect the development of newborn.
    - **Intranatal problems:** Prematurity, low birth weight, birth asphyxia, head trauma during birth, placental anomalies and umbilical cord prolapse can cause MR.

- ♦ **Postnatal problems:** Viral infections or infections like meningitis or encephalitis in newborn, kernicterus and seizure add the risk of MR.
- **Psychosocial factors**
  - Deprivation of psychological and social stimulation during infancy and childhood.
  - Poverty leading to inadequate care and nutrition in the perinatal period.
  - Cultural deprivation.
  - Child abuse.

II. Secondary Causes

Causes secondary to general medical conditions or other factors in infancy or childhood.

- Infections like meningitis, encephalitis
- Epilepsy or febrile seizure
- Poisoning with lead, insecticide, drugs or other substances (toxicity).
- Trauma

It may be seen as a coexisting problem with psychiatric conditions like autism.

General Features of Mental Retardation

- Delay in developmental milestones (motor skill, communication skill and thus socialization).
- Cognitive deficit (difficulty in understanding and following commands).
- Poor academic performance/very slow learner.
- Expressive or receptive language problems.
- Deficit in psychomotor skill.
- Difficulty in self-care.
- History of/coexisting medial or psychiatric illness (epilepsy, autism).
- Easily become irritable and frustrated with acting out behavior.

Characteristics Features of Mental Retardation

On the basis of intelligent quotient (IQ), mental retardation is classified in Table 14.1.

Table 14.1: Types of mental retardation and its characteristic features

Type of MR (IQ level)	*Characteristic features/behavior*
Mild MR (IQ 50–70) (Educable group)	• Able to live independently. Need help in stress period • Educable up to sixth grade • Able to achieve vocational skills • Able to develop social skills • Psychomotor skills are normal or may have coordination problems

Contd...

Contd...

Type of MR (IQ level)	*Characteristic features/behavior*
Moderate MR (IQ 35–49) (Trainable group)	• Do activities independently, but need supervision • Educable up to second grade • Can work in sheltered workshop • Some limitations in speech and communication, difficulty in maintaining social/peer relations • Good motor development, can do unskilled gross motor activities
Severe MR (IQ 20–34) (Dependent group)	• Elementary hygienic skills can be trained; need complete supervision • Not educable and trainable, but habit training possible • Minimal speech, needs are communicated with actions • Poor psychomotor development • Can do simple tasks with assistance
Profound MR (IQ < 20)	• Need constant help and supervision and totally dependent on caretakers • No speech and social skills • No psychomotor skills • Usually associated with physical disorders and need constant care

Diagnosis

- Detailed history collection about etiology, milestones of development, chromosomal studies and other investigations to rule out the etiology.
- Physical examination and neurological examination.
- Assessment of intelligence by the psychologist.
- $IQ = \frac{\text{Mental Age}}{\text{Chronological Age}} \times 100$

Treatment

- There is no specific treatment for MR.
- Behavior management along with environmental manipulation.
- Assess developmental needs and problems and manage them as early as possible (speech therapy, play, social skill training and training in self-care).
- Assess and treat any coexisting mental health problems like autism or attention-deficit/hyperactivity disorder (ADHD).
- Family focused interventions—parental counseling, parental education about the condition, better coping with the situation, stress management, family therapy.
- Early intervention programs for children below 3 years.
- Special schools for the moderate to severely retarded children.
- Rehabilitation/vocational training centers.

Prognosis

As there is no definite treatment for MR, prognosis also cannot be ensured. But supportive approach in the care and rehabilitation can help them to be independent according to their ability. Educable and trainable group can lead an independent life. But in problem situations, they need special concern as compared to other children.

Nursing Management

Nursing assessment must focus on detailed history collection, IQ level, behavioral manifestations, self-care ability and other strengths. Nursing diagnoses and plan should be based on the severity of problems.

Nursing Diagnoses

Table 14.2: Nursing care plan

Nursing Diagnosis	*Objectives*	*Plan of actions*
1. Risk for injury related to poor psychomotor development or impulsive behavior	Client will remain free of any injury	• Observe for activity level, signs of aggression and ability to follow instructions • Provide safe environment by: - Removing all sharp items, poisonous materials and drugs - Avoid slippery floor and keep furnishings in a well-arranged manner to prevent falls - Closely supervise as per the degree of severity and assist in activities of daily living - Keep the frequently used items nearby or within easy reach
2. Self-care deficit related to cognitive impairment and poor motor skills evidenced by inability to bath, grooming, feeding and toileting	Client participates in self-care activities	• Observe and ask about the self-care abilities and ability to follow instructions • Focus on one aspect of self-care at a time • Direct and supervise the client with simple and concrete explanations • Motivate with positive feedback for any effort for self-care and for following the instructions. Encourage independence as per client's ability • After attaining mastery in one aspect of self-care proceed with another aspect, help the client as and when needed

Contd...

Contd...

Nursing Diagnosis	*Objectives*	*Plan of actions*
3. Impaired social interaction related to limitation in speech and difficulty in social behavior evidenced by poor or dysfunctional interactions/discomfort in social interactions and situation	Client starts to interact with others	• Assess the socializing capacity of the client • Start with one tone interaction and spend more time with the client • Explain to the client about the desirable and undesirable in clear and simple language • Reinforce positive efforts and appropriate behavior by giving rewards
4. Impaired verbal communication related to developmental delay evidenced by minimal verbal skill/inappropriate verbalization or absence of speech	Client establishes trust with the nurse and communicates needs	• As far as possible, maintain consistency of staff • Anticipate and meet his/her needs, if not communicating properly • Encourage nonverbal communication and identify them with the help of family • Encourage repeated practice of communication skills both verbal and nonverbal

Prevention of Mental Retardation

As there is no specific treatment for MR, measures should be taken to prevent it:

Primary Prevention

- Some general concerns are:
  - Improvement of socioeconomic status and health promotion of people.
  - Education of the public about etiology, and to change the misconceptions about MR.
  - Promotion of good antenatal, perinatal and postnatal care
  - Prevention of malnutrition and prematurity in baby
  - Immunization of baby
  - Educate about importance of rubella vaccine to adolescent girls
  - Ensure nutrition and general health of adolescent and young females.

Antenatal Care

- Antenatal care should start in the preconception stage as provision of folic acid.
- Genetic counseling for high risk group of couples, and also for those who have family history.

- Screen for venereal disease and treat it.
- Encourage hospital delivery. Early registration and provision of antenatal care and immunization.
- Avoid exposure to radiation, occurrence of infections and use of drugs in pregnancy.
- Do antenatal visits, ultrasonography fetal monitoring.
- Care to prevent late pregnancy especially over the age of 40, through family planning measures.

Intranatal Care

- Encourage hospital delivery for good medical and nursing care in the perinatal period (to prevent obstetric complications, trauma and infections).
- Avoid prolonged labour, birth injuries and other complications.
- Immediate observation and care of new born, early detection of any defect if present.

Postnatal Care

Important aspects of care are:

- Observation
- Breastfeeding
- Screening tests—hypothyroidism
- Prevention of infection in baby
- Immunization to baby
- Exclusive breastfeeding, and good nutrition
- Physical and sensory stimulation of the child.

Secondary Prevention

- Observation and early detection of sensory or motor impairment.
- Early detection and management of underlying treatable conditions like hypothyroidism, infections, kernicterus.
- Early detection of MR helps in early intervention and rehabilitation.
- Avoid discrimination and allow them to be with the normal stream as far as possible, so that full potential in them can be facilitated.
- Children with mild MR can be educated in ordinary school.
- Those with moderate and severe degree should be educated in special schools.
- Depending on the ability, they have to be trained in self-care and vocational skills.
- Counseling to parents and other family members is very important.
- Teach the parents about adaptation to the situation, and care and rehabilitation of child.
- Encourage parents to form caregiver groups to support each other.
- In case of profound MR, hospitalization/institutionalization may be needed.

Tertiary Prevention

- Aim of this is treatment of psychological and behavioral problems to decrease the disability and to rehabilitate them as per the ability.
- Behavior modification through positive and negative reinforcement.
- Rehabilitation in different aspects as physical care, social and vocational training.
- Counseling to parents and other family members is very important.
- Teach the parents about adaptation to the situation, and care and rehabilitation of child.
- Encourage parents to form caregiver groups to support each other.
- In case of profound MR, hospitalization/institutionalization may be needed.

F80–F89: DISORDERS OF PSYCHOLOGICAL DEVELOPMENT

This group is characterized by inadequate development and problems in specific area of functioning:

- F80 - Specific developmental disorders of speech and language
- F81 - Specific developmental disorders of scholastic skills
- F82 - Specific developmental disorders of motor function
- F83 - Mixed specific developmental disorders
- F84 - Pervasive developmental disorders.

F80: SPECIFIC DEVELOPMENTAL DISORDERS OF SPEECH AND LANGUAGE

It is also known as developmental language disorder or dysphasia.

Epidemiology: In India, there is lack of prevalence studies on developmental disorders and childhood psychiatric disorders. So reliable data is not available.

Three main types of developmental disorders of speech and language are:

1. **Phonological disorder or dyslalia:** Despite normal language skills, below par accuracy in the use of speech sounds. Problems are:
   - Articulation error
   - Speech is difficult to understand for others
   - Speech sounds are substituted, distorted or omitted.
2. **Expressive language disorder:** Below par ability of expressive speech.

   Features
   - Restricted vocabulary
   - Difficulty in getting appropriate words
   - Immature grammatic use.

3. **Receptive language disorder:** Impairment in both receptive and expressive language.

   Features
   - Below par understanding of language.
   - Unable to respond to simple instructions (but deafness and pervasive developmental disorders are absent).

F81: SPECIFIC DEVELOPMENTAL DISORDERS OF SCHOLASTIC SKILLS

This can be divided as:

- **Specific reading disorder (dyslexia or developmental reading disorder)**.

  Features

  Slow in acquiring reading skills, slow reading, impairment in comprehension, letter reversal, word distortions or omissions.
- **Specific spelling disorder:** Specific reading disorder may or may not be there.

  Features

  Dysgraphia—both the ability to spell orally and to write, will be affected.
- **Specific arithmetic disorder (dyscalculia or developmental mathematic disorder):** Child shows poor arithmetic ability, that is very much below to that of the mental age.

  Features
  - Deficit in arithmetic skills of addition, subtraction, multiplication and division.
  - Inability to understand mathematical signs, concepts, calculations and mathematical tables.

F82: SPECIFIC DEVELOPMENTAL DISORDERS OF MOTOR FUNCTION

Also known as motor skills disorder, clumsy child syndrome or motor dyspraxia.

Features
- Delayed motor development.
- Clumsiness in play/work and activities in daily living (ADL).
- Inability to do fine or gross motor tasks.

Management of Specific Developmental Disorders

- Use behavioral approach in teaching, with learning theory principles
- Remedial teaching-based on specific skills

- Treat co-morbid emotional problems
- Education and counseling to parents.

F84: PERVASIVE DEVELOPMENTAL DISORDERS (PDD)

These are group of disorders that usually manifest before three years of age and characterized by abnormalities in communication and socialization and by restricted repetitive activities and interests.

DSM-V terms this as autism spectrum disorder.

Pervasive developmental disorders include childhood autism, atypical autism, Rett's syndrome, Asperger's syndrome, childhood disintegration disorder and other PDD.

AUTISTIC DISORDER

Definition: Autism is a pervasive developmental disorder characterized by withdrawal of child into self, abnormalities in communication, socialization and by restricted repetitive activities.

It is a pervasive developmental disorder characterized by withdrawal of child into self, and to a world of fantasy created by self and with restricted activities and interests that may be bizarre.

Epidemiology

- Prevalence—4-5/10000 population and is 3-4 times common in males.
- Age of onset is before 2.5 years. But rarely can occur in later childhood.
- Leo Kenner (1943) identified homogenous group of children with onset of psychosis in the first and second year of life called 'infantile autism.'
- Infantile autism has onset before the age of 2.5 years. But childhood onset autism occur in late childhood. Clinically both are almost similar. Course of illness is chronic and symptoms will continue in adulthood.

Clinical Features

Leo Kenner points out three typical features and is known as Kenner's *Autistic triad,* characteristic of infantile autism. They are:

1. Autistic aloofness
2. Speech and language disorder
3. Obsessive desire for sameness.

Common clinical features can be organized under the following headings:

- **Impairment in social and interpersonal relations (autism):** Characteristics of this are:

- Poor eye contact and lack of social smile.
- Absence of social play (child is interested in solitary play and continues it repeatedly as rowing of toys).
- Child will be aloof and not aware of presence of others.
- Not able to understand other's feelings. Treat people as inanimate objects. No emotional attachment to parents and no separation anxiety.
- No fear-even in danger situations.
- Inability in making friends.

• **Impairment in verbal and nonverbal communication**
- Lack of speech and facial expression—looks like deaf.
- Delayed speech/absence of speech/speech may not be meaningful.
- If speech is present, stereotyped speech (perseveration, echolalia), poor articulation and reversal of 'I' and 'You'.

• **Abnormal behavior pattern**
- Stereotyped behavior (clapping, head banging, lining up objects, etc.)
- Mannerisms
- Attachment to objects (objects that move or spin—like toy or fan).
- Hyperkinesis (aggression, temper tantrum).
- Routine will become an obsession and minor change itself make the child irritable.
- Abnormality in food pattern—consume excess food or eats only specific foods.
- Increased pain threshold leading to repetitive, self-injurious behavior (e.g. head banging, biting hands/arms).
- More than 50–75% of these children have mental retardation of varying degrees.
- Though there is abnormal development/mental subnormality, certain functions may remain normal (calculating ability, musical ability). It is called Idiot Savant syndrome.
- There is no hallucination, delusions or loosening of association as in schizophrenia.

Etiology of Autism

Genetic Factors

- Siblings show prevalence of 2%
- Twin studies—greater concordance in monozygotic twins.

Neurological Factors

- Central nervous system (CNS) insult in assisted labor (e.g. vacuum extraction, forceps delivery).

- Epilepsy and/or electroencephalogram (EEG) changes.
- Alteration in brain structure like increased size of ventricle.

Biochemical Factors

Elevated serotonin levels in brain.

Antenatal Causes

- Maternal bleeding after first trimester
- Use of drugs
- Mothers having asthma and allergy during pregnancy
- Birth asphyxia
- Meconium in the amniotic fluid.

Postnatal Infections

- Meningitis
- Encephalitis
- Congenital rubella
- Cytomegalovirus

Inborn Errors of Metabolism

Phenylketonuria.

Psychosocial Aspects

Kanner described the parent's features as 'refrigerator parents' who belong to high class, educated, career oriented intellectuals who are emotionally cold and aloof.

Mahler (1975)—autistic child is fixed in the presymbiotic phase of development, where the child forms a barrier from others. So the normal symbiotic relation will not occur and development of ego is inhibited.

Theory of mind—children with autism is considered as mind blind because they lack empathy.

Prognosis

- 10–20% of autistic children start to improve by the age of 4–6 years and attends in ordinary school.
- 10–20% live at home and may attend special school/training centers.
- 60% of them are unable to lead independent life and need long-term residential care.
- The children who improve also may continue with language difficulties, emotional coldness, and strange behavior.

Diagnosis

- Diagnosis is done by the age of 3 years.
- Collect a detailed history from parents.

- Do tests for genetic and neurologic problems.
- Use developmental screening to reveal autistic behavior.
- Investigate for neurologic, sensory and speech problems if MR is also present.
- Assess social behavior and language skills.

Treatment

Early intervention centers can be used for starting special care and training.

- **Pharmacotherapy:** There is no specific drug of choice for autism. But in case of aggressive, self-injurious behavior and extreme hyperactivity, drug therapy is needed. Drugs used are:
  - Haloperidol that decreases the dopamine level and thus reduces hyperactivity.
  - Risperidone is used in children of above 5 years.
  - Treatment underlying diseases if any (e.g. epilepsy).
- **Behavior therapy:**
  - A structured regular routine will be followed in home situation
  - Behavioral approach to be followed in all aspects of care
  - Training in structured classroom
  - Teach self-care skills
  - Speech therapy
  - Social skill training.
- **Education and counseling:** Education and counseling to parents for adaptation to the situation and care. Teach about behavioral approach, special schools and residential care as per their need.

Nursing Management

A detailed history collection and assessment are the foundations in nursing care.

Developmental milestones, intellectual ability, communication and social skills, specific features of autism, underlying diseases and psychosocial factors should be assessed.

Special concerns in the nursing care are:

- Individual approach in all aspects of care.
- Ensure safety by constant observation and using protective measures and safe environment.
- Alleviate anxiety in child by maintaining consistency of caregivers and by diversion activities, familiar toys, own dress materials and utensils.
- Anticipate and meet the needs without delay.
- Give positive reinforcement for any effort in communication, self-care.

- Speech therapy/and language training is very important and must get professional help.
- Child should be called by name, use simple and clear words, with clear lip movement.
- Supportive services to the parents and motivation of both the child and parents are important.

List of Nursing Diagnoses

- Risk for self-mutilation related to neurological alteration.
- Impaired social interaction related to neurological alterations, or inability to trust.
- Impaired verbal communication related to withdrawal into self, inadequate sensory stimulation or neurological alterations.
- Disabled family coping related to lack of knowledge or anxiety and poor coping skills.

Other pervasive developmental disorders are:

- **Atypical autism:** Typical features for criteria of autism are absent, especially age of onset. Mainly seen along with profound mental retardation.
- **Rett's syndrome:** Seen in girls only. Early development of the child seems to be normal, and problems starts between 7 months and 2 years of age. Acquired hand skills and speech will be lost along with deceleration of head growth. Stereotyped hand movement will be there (hand wringing).
- **Asperger's syndrome:** Sustained abnormality in social behavior, with stereotyped activities and motor mannerisms. But there is no retardation of language and cognitive development. So it is known as high functioning autism.
- **Disintegrative psychosis (Heller's syndrome):** Onset is between 3–5 years. There is deterioration and organic neurologic etiology as lipoid—degeneration of ganglia of CNS.

F90: HYPERKINETIC DISORDERS

It was first described by Heinrich Hoff in 1854. In DSM–IV TR, this was included as attention deficit hyperactive disorder (ADHD) which is a persistent pattern of inattention and/or hyperactivity and impulsivity that is more frequent and severe than is typically observed in individuals at the same age and level of development. Usually it is not diagnosed till schooling.

Epidemiology

It is 4 times more common in boys and prevalence studies are less. Course of illness is chronic and may persist to adulthood or may progress to conduct disorder.

Clinical Features

Poor Attention Span

- Easily distractible by environmental stimuli
- Not able to finish tasks due to poor attention span
- Child seems inattentive and often loses things
- Backwardness in age appropriate tasks.

Hyperactivity

- Difficulty in sitting still in a place and fidgets with hands or feet
- Excessive talk
- Interferes other's speech or activity
- Moves around in classroom.

Impulsivity

- Answer before the question is completed.
- Acts before thinking (unable to think about consequences).
- Unable to wait for their turn in sports or work.
- Highly irritable or explosive with emotional lability.

Other types that are clinically seen are:

Attention Deficit without Hyperactivity

- **Residual type:** If a person had attention deficit in the past, and diagnosed in adulthood with some residual features, it can be called residual type attention deficit disorder.
- **Hyperkinetic conduct disorder:** If hyperkinetic disorder exists with conduct disorder, it is called hyperkinetic conduct disorder.

Etiology

Though etiology is not clear, biological factors are more important.

- **Genetic factors:**
  - **Hereditary factors:** It plays an important role in etiology. Siblings of children with ADHD are more predisposed than others. Children of parents having ADHD in their childhood.
  - **Biochemical:** Abnormal levels of neurotransmitters (dopamine, norepinephrine and serotonin).

- **Problems related to pregnancy and childbirth that lead to minimal brain damage:**
  - Exposure to toxic substances like nicotine, alcohol or toxins.
  - Perinatal factors like premature birth, fetal distress, prolonged labor, birth asphyxia.
  - Postnatal factors—seizure, cerebral palsy or other trauma, infections and neurological diseases.
  - Environmental factors—lead poisoning, use of foods with preservatives and artificial flavors and colors and use of excess sugar.
- **Psychosocial factors:** Disruption in family process, and stressors like poverty, mental illness or criminality in a parent, etc.

Diagnosis

- History collection—birth and development history, including report of behavior—from parents and teachers.
- Neurological examination.
- IQ assessment to rule out mental sub-normality.
- Co-existing learning disorders.

Treatment

- CNS stimulants like dexamphetamine and methylphenidate are the commonly used drugs. These drugs stimulate the inhibitory influences on cerebral cortex by acting on the reticular activating system. Thus hyperactivity and distractibility are decreased.
- Non-stimulant medication is atomoxetine (norepinephrin reuptake inhibitor) which is a newer drug and preferred in treating attention deficit in adults.
- Parental education, counseling about condition and care are important.
- Behavior modification also must be used along with drug therapy.

List of Nursing Diagnoses

- Risk for injury related to impulsive behavior.
- Impaired social interaction related to immature behavior and inattention.
- Noncompliance with task expectations related to short attention span.
- Low self-esteem related to negative feedback from others.

F91: CONDUCT DISORDERS

Conduct disorder is characterized by repetitive and persistent pattern of conduct in which the basic rights of others are violated and important rules and regulations of the society are violated. This is more serious than the common problem behaviors in children/adolescents and may continue in adulthood as antisocial personality disorder. Features can occur before 10 years (childhood onset type) or may occur after 10 years as adolescent onset type. Conduct disorders were previously known as juvenile delinquency.

Epidemiology

This is more common in males than in females. Prevalent studies are very less.

Clinical Features

- Physical aggression with violation of rights of others—peers and family members.
- Frequent lying and stealing and fighting without guilt.
- Running away from home or school.
- Involvement in substance use, fire setting, use of weapons, breaking or destructing things.
- Cruel to other people and animals.
- Complications like substance abuse, STDs, AIDS, criminal activities including homicidal and suicidal activities.

ICD-10 points out 4 main subtypes as:

1. **Conduct disorder confined to family context.**
2. **Unsocialized conduct disorder:** It has serious underlying psychopathology.
3. **Socialized conduct disorder:** In this the individual is loyal to his or her group.
4. **Oppositional defiant disorder:** Characterized by negativistic, disobedient, a hostile behavior to authority figure and has an onset by 8 years.

Etiology

- **Genetic factor:** There is more chance to develop conduct disorder if there is a family history of it.
- **Psychosocial factors:** Poor peer relations in childhood can lead to deviance in later period.

Theory of Family Dynamics Points Out

- Rejection by the parents.
- Harsh discipline without consistency.
- Extended family.
- Absent father.

- Parental permissiveness.
- Parent with antisocial personality disorder/substance abuse.
- Marital disharmony among parents/divorce.
- Inappropriate communication pattern in the family.
- Association with delinquent groups.

Diagnosis

- History collection from parents and teachers.
- Do neurological examination.
- Investigate for neurological disorders (epilepsy).
- Assess intelligence and for learning disability.

Treatment

- There is no specific treatment for conduct disorder.
- Placement in juvenile homes/corrective institutions and management with education and behavior modifications.
- Treatment of associated problems like hyperactivity, epilepsy, mood symptoms and aggressive behavior.
- Parental education on management of child by using behavioral techniques.

F93: EMOTIONAL DISORDERS WITH ONSET SPECIFIC TO CHILDHOOD

Separation Anxiety Disorder of Childhood

This is the excess anxiety that occur when separated from the emotionally attached figure.

Features

- Unrealistic worry about possible harm to the emotionally attached persons. Child worries about some accidents and think that they may not come back.
- Refusal of sleep till the emotionally attached person comes.
- Physical symptoms while separated from emotionally attached one.
- Inappropriate fear of being alone.
- Excessive crying and apathy during separation.

Treatment

- Parental counseling to allow the child more independent rather than over protective.
- Family therapy.
- Individual counseling.
- Drug therapy (anxiolytics for short period).

Phobic Anxiety Disorder of Childhood

Simple phobic symptoms like fear of darkness, animals and school are common in childhood, but usually disappears by teenage.

Treatment

- Treatment is not needed in usual cases. A firm approach with reassurance can correct this.
- Behavior therapy—systematic desensitization is effective.

Social Anxiety Disorder of Childhood

Child shows fear of strangers that lead to avoidance of strangers and may affect the social functioning, can be treated with behavior therapy.

Sibling Rivalry Disorder

Usually seen as jealousy and competition with siblings, to get the care and affection of parents, seen few months after the arrival of younger sibling.

It is expressed as hostile and traumatic behavior to the sibling and as regressive behavior with loss of some acquired skills, e.g. loss of bladder control and starts to bed wet.

Preventive aspects like mentally preparing the elder one to accept the arrival of younger sibling during its pregnancy itself.

Take care to avoid neglect of the elder by giving adequate care and concern.

F94: DISORDERS OF SOCIAL FUNCTIONING WITH ONSET SPECIFIC TO CHILDHOOD AND ADOLESCENCE

This is a heterogeneous group of disorders that have common abnormality in social functioning that begin during developmental period.

Elective Mutism

Child shows emotionally determined selectivity in speaking. Child speaks normally in selected/familiar situations like home, but unable to speak to others.

Behavior therapy along with individual and family therapy will be effective.

F95: TIC DISORDERS

Tic is purposeless, sudden and repetitive movement that is involuntary in nature. It may be motor or vocal tics. Motor tics occur in the form of repetitive motor movements and can be:

- Simple type (e.g. shrugging of shoulders/blinking of eyes).
- Complex motor tics (e.g. jumping, squatting, copropraxia or obscene acts).
- Vocal tics occur as repetitive vocalizations and also can be simple or complex.
  - Simple vocal tics (e.g. throat clearing, sneezing, coughing)
  - Complex vocal tics (e.g. echolalia, coprolalia—says obscene words)

Multiple motor and vocal tics with more than one year duration is the characteristic feature of Gilles de la Tourette syndrome (Tourette's disorder). Treatment is with Haloperidol. If haloperidol cannot be used safely, pimozide or clonidine may be used. Behavior therapy also should be given with these.

F98: OTHER BEHAVIORAL AND EMOTIONAL DISORDERS WITH ONSET IN CHILDHOOD AND ADOLESCENCE

Nonorganic Enuresis

Repetitive voiding during day or night, at inappropriate places- which is not in accordance with child's mental age and occur without any organic basis.

Enuresis should be diagnosed only after five years.

Primary type of enuresis—here bladder control is not attained so far—till 5 years.

Secondary type—enuresis occur after a period of bladder control.

Etiology is usually psychosocial or emotional in origin (e.g. death of a parent, insecurity feelings). Before diagnosis, organic causes must be ruled out.

Management

- Fluid restriction after 8 pm.
- Bladder training.
- Wake up the child from sleep before the expected time of bedwetting.
- Supportive psychotherapy to the family.
- Drug of choice is imipramine 25–75 mg/day after the age of 6–7 years.

Nonorganic Encopresis

Repetitive passage of feces at inappropriate place and/or time without any organic cause or after bowel control is possible.

Like enuresis this also can be primary or secondary.

Secondary type usually occur between the age of 4 and 8 years and is more in males.

Etiology can be psychosocial as in enuresis, but can occur with mental retardation, autism or childhood schizophrenia.

Management is by behavior therapy with use of positive and negative reinforcement techniques. Emotional disturbance must be dealt appropriately without much delay.

SPEECH DISORDERS

- **Stuttering/Stammering**
  Characteristic features are:
  - Problem with rhythm and fluency of speech
  - Blocking of speech in between
  - Rapid repetition of words
  - Prolongation of sounds
  - Anxiety or distress associated with speech.
  - Affects 2–5% of children and common in males as compared to females.
- **Cluttering:** It is irratic and dysarrhythmic pattern of speech with jerky and rapid spurting of words and the affected person is not aware of his abnormal speech.

Treatment is with behavior modification and techniques to decrease anxiety with relaxation techniques or drugs if needed.

HABIT DISORDERS

These are unintentional, stereotyped activities that are not constructive or socially acceptable.

Common habit disorders are thumb sucking, nail biting, compulsive pulling of hair (trichotillomania), head banging, swallowing of air, teeth grinding, etc).

Treatment is by behavior modification.

CONCLUSION

There are many misconceptions that make mental illness non-acceptable, especially in childhood. Student nurse's awareness about childhood mental disorders, it is features, and etiology will help in early identification and prevention of deterioration. Effective treatment involving a combination of drug therapy, behavior therapy, play therapy and family therapy will be ideal.

BIBLIOGRAPHY

1. Ahuja N. A Short Textbook of Psychiatry (Seventh edition). New Delhi: Jaypee Brothers Medical Publishers (P) Ltd, 2011.
2. Lalitha K. Mental Health and Psychiatric Nursing: An Indian Perspective. Bangalore: VMG Book House, 2008.

3. Sadock BJ, Sadock VA, Ruiz P. Kaplan and Sadock's Synopsis of Psychiatry: Behavioral Sciences/Clinical Psychiatry (Ninth edition). Philadelphia: Wolters Kluwer, 2009.
4. Sreevani R. A Guide to Mental Health and Psychiatric Nursing (Third Edition). New Delhi: Jaypee Brothers Medical Publishers (P) Ltd, 2016.
5. Theodore DD. Textbook of Mental Health Nursing. India: Elsevier, 2015.
6. Townsend CM. Psychiatric Mental Health Nursing: Concepts of Care in Evidence-based Practice (7th edition). Philadelphia: FA Davis Company, 2012.
7. Vyas JN, Ghimire RS. Textbook of Postgraduate Psychiatry (Third edition). New Delhi: Jaypee Brothers Medical Publishers (P) Ltd, 2016.
8. WHO. Mental Health Around the World, World Health Day 2001. Geneva: WHO, 2001.
9. World Health Organization. The ICD-10 Classification of Mental and Behavioral Disorders: Clinical Descriptions and Diagnostic Guidelines. Geneva: World Health Organization, 1992.

CHAPTER 15

Community Mental Health

COMMUNITY PSYCHIATRY

Definition

Community psychiatry is defined as the provision of mental health services to the patient within their community environment with a goal to achieve full social integration.

Community mental health includes services like promotion of mental health, prevention of mental health problems, treatment and rehabilitation of psychiatric patients in the community.

Objectives of Community Mental Health Services

- Promotion of well-being and mental health
- Removing the social stigma
- Rehabilitation
- Treatment of the mentally ill using the primary health care system.

Community Mental Health Team

- Psychiatrist
- Clinical psychologist
- Psychiatric social worker
- Psychiatric nurse
- Occupational therapist
- Administrative staff to provide services.

Advantages of Community Mental Health Services

- Reduce the need for inpatient mental health services which is costly
- More accessible and acceptable to people at village level.

Barriers for Community Mental Health Services

- Stigma towards seeking mental health services
- Lack of manpower
- Lack of trained personnel, administrative and policy
- Poor coverage of rural areas
- Poor access to care

- Financial factors (expenses of travel to get services and loss of wages)
- Less priority for mental health in health policies.

Attitude, Stigma and Discrimination towards Mental Illness

Attitude about mental illness is influenced by knowledge about mental illness, experience in caring person with mental illness and media. When the society has negative attitude towards mental illness, it often result in avoidance, exclusion from daily activities and discrimination.

Stigma is defined as a group of negative attitudes and beliefs that motivate the public to fear, reject and discriminate people with mental illness. Stigma associated with mental illness is of two types:

1. **Social stigma** refers to discriminating behavior directed towards mentally ill as a result of psychiatric label.
2. **Self-stigma** refers to perception of mentally ill regarding his own illness.

Discrimination refers to unfair treatment due to a person's identity, which includes place of origin, color, creed, sex, gender identity, marital status, family status or disability, including mental disorder.

Discrimination often results in exclusion of mentally ill from education, employment and health care facilities. Stigma and discrimination worsen mental health problems and often interfere with prompt diagnosis and treatment. Consequences of stigma include poor social support, poor quality of life and low self-esteem. Stigma acts as a barrier for primary prevention, secondary prevention and tertiary prevention of mental illness.

Measures to Reduce Stigma and Discrimination to Mentally Ill

- Stop inaccurate representations of mentally ill in media.
- Mass campaigns can be arranged to educate the public regarding mental illness.
- Show empathy towards mentally ill.
- Psychoeducation to the family members regarding the etiology of mental illness.
- Conduct community awareness program focusing on:
  - Removal of stigma
  - Removal of misconceptions regarding mental illness.

COMMUNITY MENTAL HEALTH NURSING

Definition

The application of knowledge of psychiatric nursing in implementing, promoting and maintaining mental health of the people, to help in early diagnosis and care and to rehabilitate clients after mental illness (Rao, 2000).

Goals of Community Mental Health Nursing Practice

- Promote and maintain mental health
- Help to cope up with the crisis
- Educate the public regarding prevention of mental illness
- Render comprehensive psychiatric nursing services in the community.

Preventive Psychiatry

Preventive psychiatry is a branch of psychiatry that deals with health promotion, protection from mental illnesses, early diagnosis, treatment, disability limitation and rehabilitation.
There are three levels of prevention of mental illness.

Primary Prevention

Encompasses interventions to prevent mental illness and promote mental health.

Primary prevention focuses on identification of high-risk population and intervene so as to promote mental health and to reduce mental illness.

The individuals who are at risk for developing mental illness include:

- Children
- Adolescents
- Pregnant and postnatal mothers
- Old age
- Victims of violence, abuse, rape and disaster.

Primary prevention strategies for preventing the mental illness are shown in Table 15.1.

Table 15.1: Primary prevention strategies for preventing the mental illness

High-risk groups	*Primary prevention interventions*
Children	• High quality pre-school education and support visits for new parents • Adequate nutrition • Develop safe, stable and nurturing relationships between children and their parents • Educate parents regarding accident prevention • Take immunization at the appropriate time • Teachers and parents has to be educated regarding the identification of emotional and behavioral problems
Adolescents	Educational programs have to be conducted regarding: • Physical and psychological changes during puberty • Nutritional needs • Life skill education • Sexuality, pregnancy, contraception • Ill-effects of alcohol and other drugs • Counseling services available in schools

Contd...

Contd...

High-risk groups	*Primary prevention interventions*
Parenthood	• Proper antenatal care • Folic acid supplementation • Anticipatory guidance to mother and father • Encourage the couple to ventilate their worries and doubts • Educate regarding the antenatal and postnatal care
Old age	• Active involvement of the family in the care of the aged • Involvement of elderly in family gatherings • Initiate and maintenance of previous friendships • Rendering counseling services in the crisis situations • Provide education for the family members regarding the care and supporting of the aged

Role of Nurse in Primary Prevention

Nurses play an important role in primary prevention. They include:

- Provision of antenatal care to mother and educating her regarding the adverse effects of irradiation, certain drugs and prematurity.
- Encourage consumption of folic acid supplementation when planning for pregnancy.
- Encouraging for antenatal checkups and institutionalized delivery.
- Providing dietary corrections to those infants suffering from metabolic disorders.
- Training programs for mentally and physically handicapped children like blind, deaf and mute.
- Educating the teachers about the identification of emotional and behavioral problems.
- Educate the expectant mothers regarding the growth and developmental milestones.
- Provide counseling services to parents of physically and mentally handicapped, elderly and victims of violence, abuse, rape and disaster.
- Legislations and improvement of health and recreational facilities to promote mental health.

Secondary Prevention

Secondary prevention aims at early diagnosis and treatment of mental illness. Components of secondary prevention include:

- Early screening for mental illness
- Referral services
- Provision of drugs
- Crisis intervention

Nurses' Role in Secondary Prevention

- **Early diagnosis and case finding:** Community mental health nurse can conduct training programs for parents, anganwadi teachers and school teachers regarding the early identification of behavioral problems and monitoring of growth and development of children.
- **Early referral:** Teachers and public can be given information about the referral services available once the cases are identified.
- **Screening programs:** Programs for screening for mental illness can be undertaken in schools and in community.
- **Early and effective treatment:** Patients can be given drugs in district hospitals or at primary health care centers so as to improve drug compliance.
- **Mental health education:** Health education can be rendered regarding mental health promotion and prevention of mental illness at schools, primary health centers and subcenters.
- **Crisis intervention:** The person experiencing the crisis should be given timely and skillful support so as to help cope with his/her situation before physical or emotional deterioration occurs.
- **Consultation services:** Nurse can act as a consultant to deal with clients with different mental health problems.

Tertiary Prevention

Tertiary prevention aims at reducing the severity and disability associated with mental illness. Tertiary prevention mainly involves rehabilitation.

Role of Nurse in Tertiary Prevention

Family members are encouraged to participate actively in the treatment process. The nurse can organize occupational and recreational services within the hospital. Nurse can actively participate in the community rehabilitation services so that mental health services can be made accessible at door step.

Community health nurses can actively involve in programs aimed at reducing the stigma associated with mental illness.

PSYCHIATRIC REHABILITATION

Definition

It refers to a goal directed and time limited process aimed at helping an impaired person to reach the optimum mental, psychical and/or social function level.

Principles of Psychiatric Rehabilitation

- Improvement of capabilities and the competence of a person with psychiatric problems.

- Improvement of vocational outcome.
- Emphasis is on positive expectations and hope is essential.
- A deliberate increase in dependency may be the first step in the process.
- Active participation and involvement of the individual in rehabilitation.

Components of Psychiatric Rehabilitation

- Individualized approach
- Psychoeducation
- Medication monitoring
- Improvement of self-esteem
- Problem solving
- Social skill training.

Role of Nurse in Psychiatric Rehabilitation

The nurses' role in psychiatric rehabilitation includes:

- **Assessment:** The nurse has to assess the interest, abilities, interpersonal skills and limitations of the nurse. Assessment of family support, attitude and community rehabilitation agencies is also to be performed.
- **Implementation:** The mentally ill person is given social skill training, activities and vocational training. Once vocational assessment is done, based on the interests, patient is taught vocation like basket making, candle making, ornaments, stitching and cover making.

Psychoeducation is given to family regarding disease, communication skills and community rehabilitation agencies.

Types of Community Mental Health Services/Facilities

Community Mental Health Center (CMHC)

These centers render emergency services and adult, child and adolescent services. Facilities provided include medication administration, individual and family therapy and psychoeducation. CMHC may also offer rehabilitation services in the form of structured day program, vocational and residential services.

Partial Hospitalization

The patients will be in this center during the day where they will be engaged in various activities based on daily schedule. During their stay in the center, the medicines will be administered and in the evening they will return to their homes. Day care center is a type of partial hospitalization.

Examples of Day Care Centers

- SCARF (Schizophrenia Research Foundations)—Chennai
- Pakalveedu (Day Home)—Mental Health Centre, Thiruvananthapuram.

Halfway Houses

These are aftercare options for patients, who no longer need full facilities of a hospital. They need supervision for medicine administration. They are allowed adequate freedom and are able to go to work or school. The main objective of halfway homes is to promote transition from hospital to family.

Sheltered Workshop

The mentally ill patients, who cannot cope with ordinary employment, are given vocational training in a home.

Quarter Way Homes

This facility is available within the hospital itself. But there will not be regular medical rounds and most of the activities are controlled by the patients themselves.

Suicide Prevention Centers

Objective of suicide prevention centers is to create awareness among public about the warning signs of suicide and to deliver suicide prevention services.

Maithri, Kochi is a registered non-governmental organization in Kochi which offers suicide prevention services.

Primary Prevention Agencies

- Adult and youth recreational centers
- Schools
- Day care centers
- Religious places

Secondary Prevention Agencies

- Crisis centers
- Shelters (homeless, battered women, adolescents)
- Correctional community facilities
- Partial hospitalization programs
- Deaddiction centers
- Nursing homes
- Industry/work sites
- Hospices
- Assisted living facilities.

Tertiary Prevention Agencies

- Community mental health centers
- Psychosocial rehabilitation programs.

NATIONAL MENTAL HEALTH PROGRAMME (NMHP)

Mentally ill persons constitute a vulnerable section of society and are subject to discrimination in our society. National Mental Health Programme was launched by Government of India in 1982, keeping in view the heavy burden of mental illness in the community and inadequate mental health care services in the country.

India was the first developing country to formulate National Mental Health Programme. The services provided at Sakalwara, Bengaluru and Raipur Rani helped in initial development of NMHP.

Objectives of NMHP

- To ensure the availability and accessibility of minimum mental health care for all particularly to the most vulnerable and underprivileged sections of the population.
- To encourage the application of mental health knowledge in general health care and in social development.
- To promote community participation in the mental health service development and to stimulate efforts towards self-help in the community.

Role of Nurse in Mental Health Program

Liaison: Nurse can act as bridge between the public and health professional.

Educator: Community mental health nurse can conduct classes for the expectant couples, school children, parents, teachers, Anganwadi workers and lay volunteers.

Clinician: Community mental health nurse can render services aimed at providing care to the mentally ill patients at the village level. She can provide assistance in activities of daily living, conduct occupational therapy and group therapy.

Counselor: She can work as a counselor for those who are not able to cope with the situation effectively.

Coordinator: She can organise screening programs and health education programs and coordinate these activities so as to attain the objectives of mental health programs. She supervises the activities of multipurpose workers and provide training on the early detection of mental health problems.

Researcher: Involve in the various research projects of National Mental Health Programme.

CONCLUSION

Community mental health services are aimed at providing mental health care more accessible and suited to the local people. It is designed to reduce the cost of hospitalization and to favor the concept of having the mentally ill at the community level(deinstitutionalization).

BIBLIOGRAPHY

1. Ahuja N. A Short Textbook of Psychiatry (Seventh edition). New Delhi: Jaypee Brothers Medical Publishers (P) Ltd, 2011.
2. Attitudes Toward Mental Illness—Centre of Disease Control. Available from https://www.cdc.gov/hrqol/Mental_Health_Reports/pdf/BRFSS_Full%20Report.pdf Accessed on 24 May, 2017
3. Developing Community Mental Health Services—WHO South East Asia. Available from http://www.searo.who.int/entity/mental_health/documents/Accessed on 24 May, 2017.
4. Frisch N, Frisch L. Psychiatric Mental Health Nursing (Fourth Edition) Delmar Cengage Learning. New York, 2011.
5. Halter, Margaret J Varcarolis, Elizabeth M (Eds). Varcarolis' Foundations of Psychiatric Mental Health Nursing: A Clinical Approach. St Louis, MO: Elsevier, 2014.
6. Kapoor B. Textbook of Psychiatric Nursing. Delhi: Kumar Publishing House, 2014.
7. Lalitha K. Mental Health and Psychiatric Nursing. Delhi: CBS Publishers, 2009.
8. Shives RL. Basic Concepts of Psychiatric—Mental Health Nursing. Philadelphia: Lippincott Williams and Wilkins, 2008.
9. Sreevani R. A Guide to Mental Health and Psychiatric Nursing (Third Edition). New Delhi: Jaypee Brothers Medical Publishers (P) Ltd, 2016.
10. Stigma and Discrimination CMHA Ontario. Available from https://ontario.cmha.ca/documents/stigma-and-discrimination. Accessed on 24 May, 2017
11. Theodore DD. Textbook of Mental Health Nursing. India: Elsevier, 2015.
12. Townsend CM. Psychiatric Mental Health Nursing: Concepts of Care in Evidence-based Practice (7th Edition). Philadelphia: FA Davis Company, 2012.

CHAPTER 16

Psychiatric Emergencies and Crisis Intervention

DEFINITION

Psychiatric emergency is an acute disturbance of behavior, thought or mood of a patient which if untreated may lead to harm, either to the individual or to others in the environment.

Psychiatric emergency is a disturbance in thought, mood and/or action which causes sudden distress to the individual and or disability, thus requiring immediate management.

TYPES OF PSYCHIATRIC EMERGENCIES

- Suicide
- Overactivity
- Aggressive and violent behavior
- Underactivity
- Psychiatric disorder with acute onset
  - Acute psychosis
- Adverse drug reaction
- Alcohol and drug dependence
- Other psychiatric emergencies
  - Adolescent crisis
  - Rape
  - Disaster
  - Grief
  - Abuse.

SUICIDE

Suicide (deliberate self-harm) is defined as a human act of killing oneself.

Epidemiology of Suicide

Suicide occurs throughout the lifespan and it is the 17th leading cause of death in 2015 globally.

Indian Scenario

India's suicide rate was 21.1 per 100,000 people. The suicide rate in Kerala for the year 2014 is 24.9 per lakh.

Age

Suicide rates were commonly highest among older adult males, rates among young people is also increasing.

Gender

The male : female suicide ratio was 1.78 in India in 2008 and 2009.

Marital Status

Divorced, separated, widowed, and single people are more likely to commit suicide than married people.

Method of Suicide

In India, during 2009 consumption of a poison (33.6%), hanging (31.5%), self-immolation (9.2%), and drowning (6.1%) were the commonest modes of suicide.

Causes of Suicide

- **Psychiatric disorders:**
  - Major depressive disorder
  - Bipolar mood disorder
  - Schizophrenia
  - Post-traumatic stress disorder
  - Obsessive-compulsive disorder
  - Drug abuse or alcoholism
- **Medical disorders:**
  - AIDS
  - Sexually transmitted disease
  - Cancer
- **Psychosocial factors:**
  - Unemployment
  - Financial crisis
  - Marital conflicts
  - Examination failure
  - Love affairs
  - Dowry related issues

Risk Factors for Suicide

- Previous suicide attempt
- Alcohol and drug dependence
- Recent loss
- Unemployment
- Chronic medical conditions
- Poor social support.

Warning Signs of Suicide

- Talking about desire to kill oneself
- Making plans to kill oneself
- Hopelessness, worthlessness and helplessness
- Excessive use of alcohol or drugs
- Decreased sleep and/or appetite
- Social withdrawal
- Saying good-bye to loved ones.

Types of Suicide

- Altruistic suicide—suicide committed aiming at beneficial for others.
- Egoistic suicide—suicide committed as the individual's feelings and ideas are extremely different from other members of the society.
- Anomic suicide—suicide which occurs following a stressful event as the person feels that his past lifestyle is not possible in future.
- Samsonic suicide—suicide committed so as to be revengeful to others.

Nursing Management of Client with Suicidal Ideation

Nursing Diagnosis

Risk for self-directed injury related to suicidal ideations, depressive thoughts.

Objective

Client remains from self-directed injury.

Nursing Interventions

- Observe client's behavior frequently
- Observe for suicidal behaviors: Verbal statements, such as 'I am going to kill myself' or nonverbal behaviors, such as giving away valuable items.
- Determine suicidal intent and methods. Ask, 'Do you plan to kill yourself?' and 'How do you plan to do it?'
- Obtain verbal or written contract for no suicide.

- Remove all dangerous objects from client's environment.
- Maintain low level of stimuli in client's environment (low lighting, few people and low noise level).
- Keep the patient near the nurses' station.
- Avoid giving dress which has long sleeves.
- Ensure that the patient consumes medication.
- Keep medicines under safe custody.
- Administer tranquilizing medications as prescribed.

OVERACTIVE PATIENTS

Overactive patients exhibit a serious disturbance of behavior, thought and affect that makes individual unable to cope with life situations and establish interpersonal relationships. Overactive patients often are at risk of injuring himself/herself as well as others around him.

Disorders in which Overactivity is Presented

- Schizophrenia
- Mania
- Anxiety
- Delirium
- Alcohol intoxication
- Drug withdrawal.

Management of Overactive Patients

Medications—injection haloperidol (5 mg) with or without injection lorazepam (2 mg) is given.

Nursing Interventions when Dealing with Overactive Patients

- Tell the patient that you are here to help him/her.
- Always speak to the patient in simple, concise statement.
- Provide adequate space and time for the patient to talk.
- Speak in a low tone.
- Avoid arguing with the client.
- Show interest in listening and encourage the patient to talk about personal feelings and thought.
- Offer suitable and honest explanations.
- Maintain limits.
- Provide finger foods and adequate fluids.

VIOLENCE

Violence is an extreme form of aggression, such as assault, rape or murder (APA, 2017). Aggression refers to the behavior that causes harm to another person. Verbal aggression refers to psychological harm caused by the use of words. Physical aggression refers to behavior which results in physical injury to another person or property.

Causes of Violence

- Dementia
- Delirium
- Schizophrenia
- Bipolar mood disorders
- Head injuries
- Alcohol intoxication
- Antisocial and borderline personality disorders.

Symptoms of Violence

- Increasing volume of speech.
- Increased muscle tension, such as sitting on the edge of the chair.
- Tremor.
- Hyperactivity, such as pacing.
- Slamming doors or knocking over furniture.

Treatment of Violence

- Treatment focus on treating the underlying psychiatric disorders.
- Lithium is used for the treatment of bipolar disorders.
- Carbamazepine and valproate (depakote) are used to treat aggression occurring due to dementia, psychosis and personality disorders.
- Diazepam 10–20 mg can be given IV.
- Medications—injection haloperidol (5 mg) with or without injection lorazepam (2 mg) or injection phenergan (25 mg) is given.
- Physical restraint should be used as a last resort.
- Hospitalization.

Nurse's Management of a Client with Violent Behavior

Nursing Diagnosis

Risk for other-directed violence related to neurological illness, disordered thoughts, lack of impulse control, perceptual disturbances.

Nursing Interventions

- Assess the psychomotor activity of the client.
- Observe for the symptoms like increased restlessness, angry facial expressions, increased breathing and heart rate, increased speech, verbal threats or gestures, reporting anger or violent feelings.
- Provide a safe environment.

- Set limits on behavior that is destructive or adversely affects others.
- Reduce environmental stimuli.
- Provide a consistent, structured environment.
- Set realistic goals.
- Give simple direct explanations (e.g. for procedures).
- Do not argue with the client.
- Talk to the client in a low tone.
- Speak clearly and concisely.
- Encourage the client to verbalize feelings such as anxiety and anger.
- Calmly and respectfully assure the client that staff can help him in reducing the aggressive behavior.
- Explore ways to relieve tension with the client as soon as possible.
- Provide physical activity under supervision.
- Provide high calorie fluids (milk).
- Redirect the agitation and violent behavior to less dangerous activity (punching bag).
- Administer sedatives as prescribed.
- Notify the charge nurse and supervisor as early as possible about an aggressive situation.
- Apply restraints, seclusion as prescribed if needed.

Nursing Care of a Patient on Restraints

- Determine the need for restraint
- Apply restraint after it is prescribed
- Communicate to patient and family regarding the need for restraint
- Assess the restraints regularly
- Check for capillary refill and distal pulse
- Provide adequate hydration and nutrition
- Prompt documentation regarding the use of restraints.

UNDERACTIVE PATIENTS

Clinical Features of Underactive Patients

- Apathy
- Suicidal ideations
- Anorexia
- Weight loss
- Sleeplessness
- Decreased interest in activities.

Disorders in Which Underactivity is Presented

- Depression
- Catatonic stupor.

Nursing Management of Underactive Patients

- Establish a trusty nurse-patient relationship
- Maintain a calm, friendly approach
- Provide opportunity to ventilate his feelings
- Ensure adequate hydration and nutrition
- Encourage him to perform activities of daily living.

PSYCHIATRIC DISORDER WITH ACUTE ONSET

Acute Psychosis

Acute psychosis is a symptom caused by many psychiatric and medical conditions. Psychotic patients are agitated, hostile, or violent. Early signs of agitation include restlessness (pacing, fidgeting, fist clenching, posturing), irritability and decreased attention.

Management

Antipsychotics can be used for patients with or without agitation. Haloperidol can be used to treat acute psychosis. Combination of haloperidol and lorazepam is used as first-line treatment of acute agitation.

ADVERSE DRUG REACTION

Adverse drug reactions are defined as an unexpected, unintended or excessive response to a drug. Drugs which most commonly associated with adverse reactions were antipsychotics, antidepressants and mood stabilizers. The common adverse drug reaction which are psychiatric emergencies include:

- **Acute dystonia:** Characterized by involuntary, painful muscle contractions. Injection phenergan is given along with injection haloperidol to prevent dystonia.
- **Neuroleptic malignant syndrome:** Occurs as a side effect of antipsychotics. It is characterized by muscle rigidity, tachycardia, hypertension, fever and behavioral changes. Treatment includes withholding antipsychotics, supportive care and management of fever and acidosis. Bromocriptine is used as muscle relaxant.

ALCOHOL OR DRUG DEPENDENCE

Drug Withdrawal

Patient is to be kept in room with low stimuli. Physical restraints and sedation is required. Agitation is treated with lorazepam or diazepam. Hospitalization is required.

Delirium tremens occurs usually within 2–4 days after the complete stoppage of alcoholism. The classic triad of symptoms include clouding of consciousness, vivid hallucinations and tremor. Requires hospitalization. Management is with benzodiazepines, parenteral vitamin and adequate hydration.

OTHER PSYCHIATRIC EMERGENCIES

- Adolescent crisis
- Suicidal attempts, teenage pregnancy, anorexia nervosa and depression are situations which require emergency management.
- Rape
- Disaster
- Grief
- Abuse
- Child abuse are of 4 types—physical, sexual, emotional and neglect.
- Elder abuse is an intentional act or failure to act by a caregiver or another person in a relationship involving an expectation of trust that causes or creates a serious risk of harm to an older adult.

CRISIS

Definition

A sudden event in one's life that disturbs homeostasis, during which usual coping mechanisms cannot resolve the problem (Lagerquist, 2001).

Crisis is a disturbance caused by a stressful event. It usually resolves within four to six weeks.

Types

- **Maturational crisis:** Maturational crisis are developmental events which require role changes, e.g. adolescence, pregnancy, retirement.
- **Situational crisis:** These are life events that disturb the emotional health of individuals or a group, e.g. death of a loved one, pregnancy loss, divorce.
- **Adventitious crisis:** They are events that are accidental, uncommon and unexpected, e.g. disasters.

Responses to Crisis

A person's response to crisis can be categorized as physical, mental and emotional (Table 16.1).

Table 16.1: Responses to crisis

Physical	*Mental*	*Emotional*
• Nausea • Upset stomach • Tremor • Profuse sweating • Chills • Diarrhea	• Slowed thinking • Fearful thoughts • Disorientation • Memory problems	• Anxiousness • Guilt • Fear • Grief • Denial • Depression/sadness

Crisis Intervention

Crisis intervention is emergency first aid for mental health and domestic violence. The person experiencing the crisis receive timely and skillful support so as to help cope with his/her situation before physical or emotional deterioration occurs.

It is an attempt to resolve an immediate crisis when a person's usual problem-solving methods fail. The client is called on to be active in all steps of the crisis intervention process, including clarifying the problem, verbalizing feelings, identifying goals and options for reaching goals, and deciding on a plan.

Goals of Crisis Intervention

- Promotes an early recovery.
- Reduce the impact of crisis.
- Restores the adaptation.
- Reduce emotional stress and protect the client from additional stress.
- Assist the client in organizing and mobilizing resources or support systems.
- Promote adaptive family dynamics.
- Restore the client's precrisis or higher level of functioning.
- Prevent hospitalization.

Steps in Crisis Intervention (Aguilera, 1997)

- Assessment
- Planning of therapeutic intervention
- Implementation of therapeutic intervention
- Resolution of the crisis
- Evaluation.

Role of a Nurse in Crisis Intervention

Nursing Assessment

Nursing assessment should include:

- Severity of the crisis
- Perception of the crisis

- Past coping strategies
- Availability of support systems.

Nursing Diagnoses

Nursing diagnoses for clients experiencing a crisis may include the following:

- Anxiety
- Fear
- Ineffective coping
- Impaired verbal communication
- Risk for injury
- Dysfunctional grieving
- Disabled family coping.

Nursing Interventions

Environmental Manipulation

This includes those interventions that directly change the client's physical or interpersonal situation for the purpose of providing situational support or removing stress.

General Support

This includes those interventions which provide the client with the feeling that the nurse is on his side and will be a helping person. The nurse's demonstration of the therapeutic elements of warmth, acceptance, empathy and caring in addition to offering reassurance results in this type of support.

Generic Approach

This is designed to reach high risk individuals and individuals of great number in as short a time as possible.

Individual Approach

This is applicable for the diagnosis and treatment of a specific problem in a specific client. Help the client to identify the resources available in the community.

Techniques Used in Crisis Intervention

- **Catharsis:** Patient is allowed to talk about his emotions.
- **Clarification:** Patient is encouraged to give more information regarding the event.
- **Manipulation:** Patient's feelings and emotions are used for the therapy.

- **Reinforcement:** Adaptive behavior of the patient is given positive reinforcement.
- **Support of defenses:** Encourage the use of adaptive ego defense mechanism.

Modes of Crisis Intervention

- **Mobile crisis programs:** Mobile crisis units are employed to provide services to the homebound, older adult clients or individuals who live in rural areas.
- **Telephone contacts:** Suicide prevention and crisis intervention counseling centers provide telephone hotlines on a 24-hour basis.
- **Group work:** Persons with similar problem forms a group so that they can share their experiences and adopt an appropriate coping strategies.
- **Disaster response:** Nurse has an important role in dealing with the psychosocial problems of victims of disaster.
- **Victim outreach program:** Outreach programs in rural communities have been known to reduce psychiatric hospitalizations.
- **Crisis intervention centers:** Provides emergency crisis intervention to the victims of crisis.
- **Health Education:** Teaching clients, families and the community about crisis intervention and prevention are vital to promote mental health.

CONCLUSION

Psychiatric emergencies requires immediate management so as to protect the patient as well as family members. Nurses should have basic knowledge and skill in the management of psychiatric emergencies. Nurses very often has to participate in various community based crisis intervention modalities.

BIBLIOGRAPHY

1. Ahuja N. A Short Textbook of Psychiatry (Seventh edition). New Delhi: Jaypee Brothers Medical Publishers (P) Ltd, 2011.
2. American Psychiatric Association. Diagnostic and Statistical Manual of Mental Disorders (5th ed). Washington DC, 2013.
3. Halter, Margaret J Varcarolis, Elizabeth M (Eds). Varcarolis' Foundations of Psychiatric Mental Health Nursing: A Clinical Approach. St Louis, MO: Elsevier, 2014.
4. Kapoor B. Textbook of Psychiatric Nursing. Delhi: Kumar Publishing House, 2014.

5. Schultz MJ, Videbeck LS. Lippincott's Manual of Psychiatric Nursing Care Plans. Philadelphia: Wolters Kluwer, 2012.
6. Sheila Videbeck. Psychiatric Mental Health Nursing. Philadelphia: Lippincott Williams & Wilkins, 2013.
7. Shives RL. Basic Concepts of Psychiatric-Mental Health Nursing. Philadelphia: Lippincott Williams & Wilkins, 2008.
8. Sreevani R. Psychology for Nurses (Second edition). New Delhi: Jaypee Brothers Medical Publishers (P) Ltd, 2013.
9. Sreevani R. A Guide to Mental Health and Psychiatric Nursing (Third Edition). New Delhi: Jaypee Brothers Medical Publishers (P) Ltd, 2016.
10. Suicide rates—Kerala State Mental Health Authority. Available from www.ksmha.org/suicide.htm.
11. Theodore DD. Textbook of Mental Health Nursing. India: Elsevier, 2015.
12. Townsend CM. Nursing Diagnoses in Psychiatric Nursing Care Plans and Psychotropic Medications (8th Edition). Philadelphia: FA Davis Company, 2011.
13. Townsend CM. Psychiatric Mental Health Nursing: Concepts of Care in Evidence-based Practice (7th edition). Philadelphia: FA Davis Company, 2012.
14. Violence Prevention Home Page—CDC Available from https://www.cdc.gov/violenceprevention.
15. Vyas JN, Ghimire RS. Textbook of Postgraduate Psychiatry (Third edition). New Delhi: Jaypee Brothers Medical Publishers (P) Ltd, 2016.
16. WHO|Suicide data Available from www.who.int/mental_health/prevention/suicide/suicideprevent/en.
17. World Health Organization. The ICD-10 Classification of Mental and Behavioral Disorders: Clinical Descriptions and Diagnostic Guidelines. Geneva: World Health Organization, 1992.

CHAPTER 17 Forensic Psychiatry

Forensic psychiatry is the branch of psychiatry which deals with relation of legal principles to mental disorders. Forensic psychiatry includes:
- Criminal responsibility
- Civil responsibility
- Laws relating to psychiatric disorders
- Rights of mentally ill
- Admission procedures of mentally ill.

CRIMINAL RESPONSIBILITY

In 1843, Daniel McNaughton attempted an assassination on the Prime Minister, and accidentally shot the secretary of the Prime Minister. McNaughton suffered from paranoia and delusions of persecution. After trial, McNaughton was acquitted of his actions because he was deemed 'insane' and he was not responsible for his actions. McNaughton rule states that at the time of crime if the person has disease of the mind, then he is not guilty of that crime.

In India, Section 84 of Indian Penal Code states that nothing is an offence which is done by a person who at the time of crime is of unsound mind and does not know the nature of his act.

CIVIL RESPONSIBILITY

Marriage

Marriage between two individuals of which one is of unsound mind at the marriage is considered null and void. Unsound mind continuously for a period of more than 2 years can be a ground for obtaining divorce.

Management of Property

The court appoints a manager to take care of the property of a person who is found to have an unsound mind after inquisition.

Testamentary Capacity

Refers to the ability of a person to make a valid will. The person should be a major and possess a sound mind to make a valid will.

Right to Vote

A person cannot vote or contest for election if he is having unsound mind.

LAWS RELATING TO PSYCHIATRIC DISORDERS

Indian Lunacy Act (ILA, 1912)

This act is derived from English Lunacy Act, 1890 and has 8 chapters. Indian Lunacy Act resulted in the establishment of new asylums and improvement in existing conditions of asylums.

Chapter I: Short Title and Extent

This chapter gives the definition of terms. Asylum means mental hospital for lunatics established or licensed by the Central Government or any State Government. Lunatic means an idiot or a person of unsound mind.

Chapter II: Reception of Lunatics

This chapter deals with the admission of a lunatic.

Chapter III: Care, Treatment and Visitors

This chapter explains the discharge of lunatics and appointment of visitors. It specifies that State Government shall appoint not less than three visitors for every asylum, one of whom at least shall be a medical officer.

Chapter IV: Proceedings in Lunacy in Presidency-towns

This chapter provides guidelines for undertaking inquiries regarding the lunatic. On inquisition if it is found that the person to whom the inquisition relates is of unsound mind and is incapable of managing his affairs, the Court may make such orders for the management of the estate of the lunatic including proper provision for the maintenance of the lunatic.

Chapter V: Proceedings in Lunacy outside Presidency-towns

A manager appointed can continue only so long as the lunatic is alive. When the lunatic dies, the lunacy jurisdiction comes to an end and the Court must pass some order about the property in the hands of the manager.

Chapter VI: Establishment of Asylums

State Government may establish or licence the establishment of asylums for the treatment of lunatics.

Chapter VIII: Rules

Rules to be formulated by the state government for the care of lunatics is discussed in this chapter.

Mental Health Act, 1987

Mental Health Act was drafted by the Indian Parliament in 1987 and it came into existence in April 1993. The Mental Health Act was aimed to consolidate and amend the law relating to treatment and care of mentally ill persons regarding their property.

Objectives of Mental Health Act

- Regulates the admission of mentally ill.
- Protects the society from mentally ill.
- Establish and maintain mental hospitals.
- Provide legal aid to mentally ill.

Chapters of Mental Health Act

Mental health act, 1987 has 10 chapters (Table 17.1).

Table 17.1: Chapters of Mental Health Act, 1987

Chapters	*Titles*
I	Preliminary
II	Mental Health Authorities
III	Psychiatric hospitals and psychiatric nursing homes
IV	Admission and detention in psychiatric hospital or psychiatric nursing home
V	Inspection, discharge, leave of absence and removal of mentally ill persons
VI	Judicial inquisition regarding alleged mentally ill person possessing property, custody of his person
VII	Liability to meet cost of maintenance of mentally ill persons
VIII	Protection of human rights of mentally ill persons
IX	Penalties and procedures
X	Procedures

Chapter I: Preliminary—short title, extent and terminology

This chapter deals with definition of terminologies. The Act replaces the term 'luantic' with 'mentally ill person' and defines it as 'a person who is in need of treatment by reason of any mental disorder other than mental retardation'.

Other terms which are defined in this chapter are psychiatric hospital, psychiatric nursing home and psychiatrist.

Chapter II: Mental Health Authorities

Authority for mental health has been established by the Central Government and the State Government to supervise the psychiatric hospitals, psychiatric nursing homes and other Mental Health Agencies under the control of the Central Government and State Government.

Chapter III: Psychiatric hospitals and nursing homes

The Central Government or the State Government may, within the limits of its jurisdiction, establish or maintain psychiatric hospitals or psychiatric nursing homes for the admission, treatment and care of mentally ill persons.

Chapter IV: Admission and detention in psychiatric hospital, or psychiatric nursing home

This chapter deals with procedures for the admission and discharge of mentally ill person. It includes different sections which explain the method of admission. Some of them are shown in Table 17.2.

Table 17.2: Different sections which explain the method of admission

Section	*Type of admission*	*Description*
Section 15	Admission on voluntary basis (Major)	Any person (major) may request for admission to the medical officer. On receiving the request, medical officer shall make enquiry within 24 hours and if found mentally ill, he will be admitted
Section 16	Admission on voluntary basis (Minor)	Guardian make a request to the medical officer for admission for a minor
Section 19	Admission of mentally ill persons under certain special circumstances	Any mentally ill person who does not, or is unable to, express his willingness for admission as a voluntary patient, may be admitted and kept as an inpatient in a psychiatric hospital on an application made in that behalf by a relative or a friend of the mentally ill
Section 24	Procedure on production of mentally ill person	On production of mentally ill person (e.g. wandering or neglected mentally ill person) before magistrate. The magistrate instruct the medical officer to examine and if found mentally ill, issues a reception order so as to admit the patient in a psychiatric hospital
Section 27	Admission of mentally ill prisoner	Mentally ill prisoner is admitted to mental hospital on the order of court

Chapter V: Inspection, discharge, leave of absence and removal of mentally ill persons

The State Government or the Central Government shall appoint for every psychiatric hospital and every psychiatric nursing home, not less than five visitors, of whom at least one shall be a medical officer, preferably a psychiatrist and two social workers. Inspection has to be done at least once in every month.

This chapter also deals with rules related to discharge of mentally ill. The procedure for discharge is included in different sections (Table 17.3).

Table 17.3: Different sections which explain the discharge of mentally ill

Section	*Type of discharge*	*Description*
Section 18 (Chapter IV)	Discharge on voluntary basis	Medical officer can issue an order for discharge based on the recommendation of two psychiatrists on behalf of the request made by major or guardian for minor
Section 40	Order of discharge by medical officer in charge	Medical officer issues discharge based on the recommendation of two medical practitioners
Section 41	Discharge of mentally ill persons on application	Any person detained in a psychiatric hospital or psychiatric nursing home under an order shall be discharged based on an application to the medical officer in charge
Section 42	Order of discharge on the undertaking of relatives or friends, for due care of mentally ill	Relatives make a request to the medical officer in charge for discharge. A bond has to be executed

Leave of Absence (Section 45)

An application for leave of absence on behalf of any mentally ill person (not being a mentally ill prisoner) undergoing treatment as an inpatient in any psychiatric hospital or psychiatric nursing home may be made by the husband or wife to the medical officer-in-charge. Each application shall be accompanied by a bond stating that the mentally ill will be given proper care and they will be brought back to psychiatric hospital or psychiatric nursing home. Leave of absence granted shall not exceed 60 days.

Chapter VI: Judicial inquisition regarding alleged mentally ill person possessing property, custody of his person

Deals with judicial inquisition regarding the mentally ill person, possession of property, their custody and management of property. An order can be issued by the court for the appointment of a guardian, if it feels that the alleged mentally ill person is incapable of looking himself and his property. But if the court feels that the person is only incapable of looking after his property, an order is issued to appoint a manager.

Chapter VII: Liability to meet cost of maintenance of mentally ill persons

This chapter states that State Government has the liability to meet the cost of maintenance of mentally ill person detained in psychiatric hospitals or nursing homes.

Chapter VIII: Protection of human rights of mentally ill persons

The following rules are included for the protection of human rights of mentally ill:

- No mentally ill person shall be subjected, during treatment, to any indignity.
- No mentally ill person, under treatment, shall be used for the purposes of research, unless such research is of direct benefit to him.
- No letters or communication sent by or to a mentally ill person shall be detained or destroyed.

Chapter IX: Penalties and procedures

Chapter IX deals with the procedures for the establishment of psychiatric hospitals and nursing homes and the penalties if not followed.

Chapter X: Procedures

This chapter provide clarification regarding certain procedures to be followed by medical officer.

Mental Health Care Act, 2017

An Act of Parliament was passed on 7th April, 2017 to provide for mental health care and services for persons with mental illness and to protect, promote and fulfill the rights of such persons during delivery of mental health care and services and for matters connected. This Act has replaced Mental Health Act, 1987. Chapters of Mental Health Care Act, 2017 are shown in Table 17.4.

Table 17.4: Chapters of Mental Health Care Act, 2017

Chapters	*Titles*
I	Preliminary
II	Mental illness and capacity to make mental health care and treatment decisions
III	Advance directive
IV	Nominated representative
V	Rights of persons with mental illness
VI	Duties of appropriate government
VII	Central mental health authority
VIII	State mental health authority
IX	Finance, accounts and audit
X	Mental health establishments
XI	Mental health review boards
XII	Admission, treatment and discharge
XIII	Responsibilities of other agencies
XIV	Restriction to discharge functions by professionals not covered by profession
XV	Offences and penalties
XVI	Miscellaneous

Narcotic Drugs and Psychotropic Substances Act, 1985 (NDPS Act)

Formulated by the Parliament of India. Amendment of the NDPS Act has been made in 1988, 2001 and 2014. This Act prohibits a person to produce/manufacture/cultivate, possess, sell, purchase, transport, store, and/or consume any psychotropic drug or narcotic.

No person shall engage in or control any trade whereby a narcotic drug or psychotropic substance is obtained outside India and supplied to any person outside India.

Any person who manufactures, possesses, sells, purchases, transports, imports any manufactured drug or psychotropic drug shall be subjected for rigorous imprisonment for not be less than ten years but which may extend to twenty years and shall also be liable to fine which shall not be less than one lakh rupees but may extend to two lakh rupees.

For repeat offence, he shall be subjected for rigorous imprisonment for not be less than fifteen years but which may extend to thirty years and shall also be liable to fine which shall not be less than 1.5 lakh rupees but may extend to three lakh rupees.

Rights of Mentally Ill

Rights of mentally ill person are shown in Table 17.5.

Table 17.5: Rights of mentally ill person

- The right to wear their own clothes
- The right to keep and use their own personal articles
- The right to have own individual storage space for their private use
- The right to see visitors every day
- The right to have reasonable access to telephones, both to make and to receive calls
- The right to have ready access to letter-writing materials
- The right to refuse electroconvulsive therapy
- The right to spend reasonable money for canteen expenses and small purchases
- The right to manage and dispose of property
- The right to execute wills
- The right to hold civil service status
- The right to treatment in the least restrictive setting

Legal Responsibilities of a Nurse in the Care of Mentally Ill

Psychiatric nurses must be aware of patient's rights, criminal, civil responsibilities and admission discharge procedures of mentally ill patients.

Nurse's Responsibility in Admission

The role of nurse in admitting mentally ill patient is as follows:

- Orient the patient to ward routines—daily activities, medication, meals, visiting time.
- Perform a head to foot assessment.

- Collect history and do mental status examination.
- Meet the needs of the patient.
- Alleviate the anxiety/fear of the patient.
- Closely observe the patient if he/she has suicidal ideations.
- Maintain good nurse-patient relationship.
- Provide a safe and therapeutic environment.
- Administer the medications as prescribed.
- Provide adequate information.
- Document the admission procedure.

Nurse's Responsibility in Discharge

- Provide education regarding medication.
- Reinforce the need for regular follow up and importance of adherence to therapeutic regime.
- Document the discharge procedure and return the file.

Ensure Confidentiality

American Nurses Association advocates protecting confidentiality of patients. Information related to the mentally ill should not be disclosed.

Obtaining an Informed Consent

Informed consent has to be obtained from mentally ill patients with due consideration to their soundness of mind, intelligence and comprehension ability. Informed consent should include nature of the treatment, risk and benefit of treatment.

Avoid Negligence

Negligence is doing something which a reasonably prudent person would not do, or the failure to do something which a reasonably prudent person would do, under the circumstances similar to those shown by the evidence.

Intentional Torts

Intentional torts are when others interfere with others' privacy, property and interests. Some of intentional torts are:

Battery: Refers to an intentional and wrongful physical contact with another person without that person's consent.

Assault: Assault is the intentional act of making someone fear that one will cause them harm.

False imprisonment: An intentional act of preventing one person from moving about.

Defamation: Written or spoken communication, that is untrue and that injures reputation of another.

Maintain Standards of Nursing Care

American Nurses Association has put forth Psychiatric Mental Health Nursing Practice standards. Psychiatric Mental Health Nurses has to follow these standards to provide quality care to mentally ill.

Documentation

Nurses should document assessment data, treatment correctly and the medical records should be kept under safe custody as these are legal documents.

CONCLUSION

Psychiatric Mental Health Nurses should be aware of the legal aspects pertaining to psychiatric patients, for safeguarding the patients as well as society.

BIBLIOGRAPHY

1. Ahuja N. A Short Textbook of Psychiatry (Seventh edition). New Delhi: Jaypee Brothers Medical Publishers (P) Ltd, 2011.
2. Halter, Margaret J Varcarolis, Elizabeth M (Eds). Varcarolis' Foundations of Psychiatric Mental Health Nursing: A Clinical Approach. St Louis, MO: Elsevier, 2014.
3. Kapoor B. Textbook of Psychiatric Nursing. Delhi: Kumar Publishing House, 2014.
4. Lalitha K. Mental Health and Psychiatric Nursing. Delhi: CBS Publishers, 2009.
5. Mental Healthcare Act, 2017-PRS. Available from www,psrindia.org/.../Mental%20Health/Mental%20Healthcare%20Healthcare%20Act,%20 2017.pdf. Accessed on 16 June 2017.
6. Sreevani R. A Guide to Mental Health and Psychiatric Nursing (Third Edition). New Delhi: Jaypee Brothers Medical Publishers (P) Ltd, 2016.
7. Theodore DD. Textbook of Mental Health Nursing. India: Elsevier, 2015.
8. Vyas JN, Ghimire RS. Textbook of Postgraduate Psychiatry (Third edition). New Delhi: Jaypee Brothers Medical Publishers (P) Ltd, 2016.

Appendices

APPENDIX 1: MENTAL HEALTH NURSING FORMAT FOR HISTORY AND MENTAL STATUS EXAMINATION

IDENTIFICATION DATA

Name
Age
Gender
Education
Occupation
Income
Religion
Address
Source of referral

Informant Details

Name:
Age:
Relationship to the patient:
Familiarity and duration of stay:
Adequacy and reliability of the information:

PRESENTING CHIEF COMPLAINTS WITH DURATION

Patient's Version

Should be recorded in patient's own words.

Informant's Version

Record the complaints with its duration in a chronological order.

HISTORY OF PRESENT ILLNESS

- **Mode of Onset:** Abrupt (within hours), acute (within 1 week), subacute (1 – 2 weeks), insidious (few weeks – few months), chronic (more than 6 months).

- **Duration:** (Weeks/months/years)
- **Course:** Episodic/continuous/fluctuating/deteriorating/improving
- **Precipitating factors/aggravating factors:** Physical/psychosocial/pharmacological factors.
- **Description:** When was the client apparently normal, chronological account of client's abnormal behavior during present episode.
- **Associated disturbances:** In biological, occupational, social and interpersonal dimensions.

PAST HISTORY

History of Past Psychiatric Illness

- Total duration of illness
- Describe each episode including nature and duration of symptoms, treatment received and duration of hospitalization.

History of Past Medical-Surgical Illness

Fever/trauma/headache/vomiting/confusion/disorientation/memory disturbances/neuropathy/head injury/meningitis/encephalitis/epilepsy/typhoid/TB/syphilis.

FAMILY HISTORY

Genogram (In Three Generation)

- Describe each member of family with age, education, occupation, health status.
- Consanguinity between parents.

Details of Family Functioning

Type of family, socioeconomic status, other relevant details.

History of Illness in the Family

History of psychiatric illnesses, delinquency, personality problems, suicide, substance abuse, epilepsy and mental retardation.

PERSONAL HISTORY

Birth and Early Development

- **Antenatal period:**
  - Uneventful/eventful
  - Include details about mother's health/pregnancy induced hypertension/diabetes mellitus/bleeding/infections

- **Intranatal period:**
  - Birth—full term/premature/postmature
  - Delivery normal/instrumental/cesarean
  - Place of delivery
  - Birth cry—immediate/delayed
  - Birth defects—if any
- **Postnatal period:**
  - Postnatal complications—cyanosis/convulsions/jaundice
  - Postpartum psychosis for mother/any other.

Childhood History

- **Infancy:** Developmental milestones (motor, adaptive, developmental, social)—normal/delayed.
- **Behavior and emotional problems:** Presence of sleep disturbances/thumb-sucking/nail-biting/temper tantrums/bed-wetting/stammering/tics/mannerisms/attention deficits/impulsivity/disobedience/fears/worrying/lack of self-confidence/attention seeking behaviors.
- **Home atmosphere in childhood and adolescence:** Broken home/stepparents/adopted sibling.
- **Attitude towards the parents**
- **Emotional problems during adolescence:** Running away from home/delinquency/smoking/drug taking/truancy/any other.

Educational History

- Age at the beginning of formal education
- Maximum educational status achieved
- Any failures, reason for failure
- Academic and extracurricular achievements
- Attitude/relationship with teachers
- **School phobia:** yes/no
- Disciplinary problems
- Discontinuation/change of school
- Relationship with playmates

Occupational History

- Age at starting the work
- Jobs held in chronological order
- Frequent changes in jobs
- Reason for changes
- Present job
- Job satisfaction

- Promotions/awards
- Relationship with colleagues, superiors and subordinates.

Menstrual History

- Age at menarche and reaction to menarche
- Regularity of cycles and duration of flow
- Associated physical and psychological symptoms to current cycle
- Abnormalities if any
- Last menstrual period.

Sexual History

- Age at appearance of secondary sexual characters
- Anxiety related to puberty changes source/level of knowledge regarding sex.
- History of sexual abuse.
- Premarital/extramarital sexual relations.

Marital History

- **Type of marriage:** Self-choice/arranged
- Age at time of marriage
- Age/education/occupation/health of the partner at marriage
- **Interpersonal and sexual relations with spouse:** Satisfactory/unsatisfactory.

Obstetrical History

- Number of children
- Any abnormalities associated with pregnancy, delivery and puerperium.
- Age at menopause and associated problems, if any.

PREMORBID PERSONALITY

- **Interpersonal relationships:** Introvert/extrovert
- **Attitude to self:** positive/negative, selfish/thought to others
- **Attitude to others:** positive/negative, selfish/thought to others
- **Attitude to work and responsibility:** Decision-making power, acceptance of responsibility, flexibility
- **Use of leisure time:** Hobbies/interest/intellectual activity/ energetic/ sedentary.
- **Predominant mood:** Optimistic/pessimistic/stable/fluctuating/ cheerful/despondent.
- **Reaction to stressful events**

- **Religious belief and moral attitudes**
- **Habits**
  - Eating pattern
  - Elimination
  - Sleep
  - Use of drug, tobacco, alcohol, other psychoactive substances.

Psychoactive Substance Use History

- Age at first use
- Cause of first use
- First experience with psychoactive substance
- History of tolerance
- History of craving
- History of dependence
- History of withdrawal symptoms
- Period of longest abstinence from psychoactive substance
- Reason for restarting
- Reason for excessive consumption
- Maintaining factors
- Money spent for daily use
- History of other substance use.

Physical Examination

Include head to foot assessment and system wise examination.

MENTAL STATUS EXAMINATION

Date:
Time:

General Appearance

- **Appearance:** Looks same as/younger than/older than that of stated age
- **Body built:** Ectomorphic/mesomorphic/endomorphic
- **Hygiene and grooming:** Normal/shabbily dressed/overdressed/idiosyncratically dressed
- **Mode of entry:** Came willingly/persuaded/brought using physical force
- **Posture:** Normal/catatonic/odd
- **Gait:** Steady/unsteady
- **Facial expression**
- **Eye to eye contact:** Maintained/difficult/not maintained
- **Gesture:** Normal/exaggerated/odd

- **Rapport:** Spontaneously established/maintained/difficult to establish/could not establish
- **Attitude towards the examiner:** Cooperative/noncooperative/guarded/evasive/hostile/haughtiness/apathetic
- **Hallucinatory behaviors**
- **Psychomotor activity:** Increased/decreased/normal
- **Other disorders:** Tics/stereotyped movements, mannerisms and gestures, restlessness and agitation, aggressiveness, rigidity, echopraxia, negativism.

Speech

Speech sample of client (ask the patient to talk about a neutral topic—weather, festivals, famous personalities).

- **Initiation:** Spontaneous/speaks when spoken to/minimal/mute
- **Reaction time:** Normal/delayed/shortened/difficult to assess
- **Rate:** Normal/slow/rapid
- **Amount/productivity:** Normal/decreased/increased
- **Tone (loudness):** Normal/decreased/increased
- **Prosody of speech:** Maintained/not
- **Relevance:** Fully relevant/sometimes off target/irrelevant
- **Coherence:** Fully coherent/loosening of associations
- **Others:** Rhyming/punning/echolalia/perseveration/neologism/clang association.

Thought

- **Form:** Normal/thought disorder: neologism/flight of ideas/clang association/glossolalia/word salad (*specify with a sample of speech*).
- **Stream:** Normal/abnormal-loosening of association/circumstantiality/tangentiality/thought block/retardation of thinking/perseveration.
- **Content:** Delusions—grandiose/persecutory/nihilistic/jealousy/infidelity/love/somatic/hypochondriacal/ poverty/guilt.
- Depressive ideations (ideas of worthlessness/hopelessness/helplessness)/guilt/suicidal ideations/phobias.
- **Possession:** Obsessions and compulsions, thought alienation—thought insertion/thought control/thought broadcasting/thought withdrawal.

Emotion

- Mood (longitudinal assessment)
- **Subjective:** What the patient says
- **Objective:** Happiness/sadness/anxious/depressed/euthymic/elated

- Affect
- **Range:** (of affective response)—Normal/constricted/blunted/flat

Perception

- **Hallucinations:** Visual/auditory/tactile/olfactory/gustatory/pain/deep sensations
- Illusion
- Depersonalization
- Derealization.

Cognitive Functions

- **Consciousness:**
- **Orientation:** Time:
  Place:
  Person:
- **Memory:**
  - *Immediate:* Digit span test/recall name of 3 unrelated objects
  - *Recent:* Recent happenings/last meal/visitors, etc.
  - *Remote:* Recall of personal or impersonal events—date of birth/date of marriage/names and number of family members/year of completing education.

  (*Always attempt to verify from the informant*)
- **Attention:** Normally aroused/aroused with difficulty
  - *Tests:* Digit span test—digit forward and backward test/weekdays /month/letters of the word W-O-R-L-D forward and backward
  - Digit forward test:

    1 - 4
    2 - 5 - 8
    9 - 2 - 5 - 1
    6 - 2 - 8 - 3 - 7
  - Repeat with different digits if patient make mistake—1 - 9 - 4 - 7 - 3
  - Digit backward test:

    4 - 1
    8 - 5 - 2
    1 - 5 - 2 - 9
    7 - 3 - 8 - 2 - 6
- **Concentration**
  - *Tests:* Serial subtraction

100–7 [120 sec]
40–3 [60 sec]
20–1 [15 sec]
(Note the answers and time taken)

  - *Inference:* Normally sustained/distractible

- **Intelligence:**
  - *General fund of information:* Relevant to patient's education/occupation
  - *Arithmetic ability:* All the 4 mathematical operations, (+, ÷, −, ×)
  - *Inference:* Intelligence is below average/average/normal
- **Abstract thinking:**
  - *Proverb test*
  - *Similarity and dissimilarity*
- **Judgment**
  - *Personal* (Q: what is your future plan?)
    - *Inference:* Intact/impaired
  - *Social:* (how the patients behave in a social situation with other patients and relatives and respond to the examiner)
    - *Inference:* Intact/impaired
  - *Test:* Letter test/fire test
    - *Inference:* Intact/impaired
- **Insight:** Check the patient's level of awareness of his illness.
  - Grading of Insight:
    - Grade I: Complete denial of illness.
    - Grade II: Slight awareness of being sick, need help but denying it at the same time.
    - Grade III: Awareness of being sick but blaming it on an external factors or organic factors.
    - Grade IV: Awareness that illness is due to something unknown in patient.
    - Grade V: Intellectual insight
    - Grade VI: True emotional insight.

Physical Examination

Summary

Diagnostic formulation.

APPENDIX 2: FORMAT—PROCESS RECORDING

Name of the Client
Age
Ward No
Marital status
Occupation
Date of Admission

Chief Complaints

- According to client
- According to informant

Introductory Remarks

- Appearance of the patient including his behavior:
- Nurse's feelings and thoughts prior to interaction:
- Setting of the interaction:

Date: Time and duration:

Objectives of this Interaction

What the nurse said and did	*What the patient said and did*	*Therapeutic communication technique used*	*Analysis of the patient's response*

Summary

APPENDIX 3: FORMAT FOR NURSING CARE PLAN—MENTAL HEALTH NURSING

- **Identification data**
  Name
  Age
  Gender
  Education
  Occupation
  Income
  Religion
  Address
  Source of referral
  Informant details
  Name:
  Age:
  Relationship to the patient
  Familiarity and duration of stay
  Adequacy and reliability of the information.
- **Presenting chief complaints with duration**
- **History of present illness**
- **Past history**
  - History of past psychiatric illness
- **Family history**
- **Personal history**
- **Premorbid personality**

Physical examination

Include head to foot assessment and system wise examination

Mental status examination (MSE)

Treatment

List of Nursing Diagnoses

Nursing Care plan

Assessment	*Nursing diagnosis*	*Objective*	*Plan of action*	*Implementation*	*Evaluation*

Psychoeducation
Conclusion

APPENDIX 4: FORMAT FOR CARE STUDY/CLINICAL PRESENTATION—MENTAL HEALTH NURSING

- **Identification data**
  Name
  Age
  Gender
  Education
  Occupation
  Income
  Religion
  Address
  Source of referral

  Informant details
  Name:
  Age:
  Relationship to the patient:
  Familiarity and duration of stay:
  Adequacy and reliability of the information:
- **Presenting chief complaints with duration**
- **History of present illness**
- **Past history**
  - History of past psychiatric illness
- **Family history**
- **Personal history**
- **Pre-morbid personality**

Physical Examination

Include head to foot assessment and system wise examination

Mental status examination (MSE)

Disease aspect
- Definition
- Epidemiology
- Etiology

Book picture	*Patient picture*

- Classification
- Clinical features

Book picture	*Patient picture*

- Diagnosis

Book picture	*Patient picture*

- Management

Book picture	*Patient picture*

(Include drug file)

Nursing Management

- List of nursing diagnoses
- Nursing care plan

Assessment	*Nursing diagnosis*	*Objective*	*Plan of action*	*Implementation*	*Evaluation*

Psychoeducation

Progress Notes

Conclusion

APPENDIX 5: FORMAT FOR PSYCHOEDUCATION

Topic: Group:
Time:
Venue:

Method of teaching:

AV Aids:

Previous level of knowledge:

General objective:

Specific objectives:

Objective	*Time*	*Content*	*AV aids*	*Teaching and learning activity*	*Evaluation*

Summary

Recapitulation

Bibliography

APPENDIX 6: MINI MENTAL STATE EXAMINATION (MMSE)

Patient's Name: Date:

Instructions: Ask the questions in the order listed. Score one point for each correct response within each question or activity.

Maximum score	*Patient's score*	*Questions*
5		'What is the year? Season? Day of the week? Month?
5		'Where are we now: State? Country? Town/City? Hospital? Floor'
3		The examiner names three unrelated objects clearly and slowly, then asks the patient to name all three of them. The patient's response is used for scoring. The examiner repeats them until patient learns all of them, if possible. Number of trials:......
5		'I would like you to count backward from 100 by sevens' (93,86,79, 65....). Stop after five answers. Alternative: 'Spell WORLD backwards'(D-L-R-O-W).
3		'Earlier I told you the names of three things. Can you tell me what those were'?
2		Show the patient two simple objects, such as wristwatch and a pencil and ask the patient to name them.
1		'Repeat the phase: 'No ifs, ands or buts'.
3		'Take the paper in your right hand, fold it in half and put it on the floor'. (The examiner gives the patient a piece of blank paper)
1		'Please read this and do what it says'. (Written instruction is 'Close your eyes').
1		'Make up and write a sentence about anything'. (This sentence must contain a noun and a verb).
1		'Please copy this picture'. (The examiner gives the patient a blank piece of paper and asks him/her to draw the symbol below. All 10 angles must be present and two must intersect.
30		**Total**

(Adapted from Rovner and Folstein, 1987)

SAMPLE OF PSYCHIATRIC ASSESSMENT

PSYCHIATRIC HISTORY

Identification Data

Name	:	Mrs X
Age	:	48 years
Gender	:	Female
Education	:	4th std
Occupation	:	nil
Income	:	₹1500
Religion	:	Hindu
Address	:	Thiruvananthapuram
Ward	:	10

Informant details

Name	:	Mrs Y
Age	:	70 Years
Relationship to the patient	:	Mother

Familiarity and duration of stay : Familiar, 48 years

Adequacy and reliability of the information: Adequate and reliable

Presenting Chief Complaints with Duration

Patient's version: 'I have no problem. My relatives brought me to here for harming me.'

Informant's version:

Reduced sleep	× 2 weeks
Reduced appetite	× 1 week
Increased religiosity	× 1 week
Increased talk	× 1 week
Singing songs	× 4 days
Violent behavior	× 1 day

History of Present Illness

Mode of onset: Acute

Course: Episodic

Precipitating factors/aggravating factors: Pharmacological factors—drug noncompliance for 1 month.

Description: Mrs X was apparently normal 2 weeks back. The symptoms started as reduced sleep, slept only a few hours, reduced appetite. She had increased speech and singing religious songs and going to the temple more frequently. She used to quarrel with her husband without any reason and use abusive words towards others especially to the neighbors and throws stones to their houses. As she showed violent behavior towards others, her husband and other relatives brought her to medical college hospital and admitted in ward ....

Associated Disturbances

In biological—reduced sleep and decreased need for food intake, neglect personal hygiene.

Social and interpersonal dimensions—increased sociability and irritable sometimes to others.

Past History

History of Past Psychiatric Illness

- **Total duration of illness:** 1 year
- **Initial onset in detail:** She has episodic psychiatric illness since 2016. The first onset of illness occurred after the death of her brother and the symptoms started as decreased appetite, decreased sleep, reduced social interaction, remain confined in a room, not taking care of herself, withdrawn behavior and had suicidal ideations. So her relatives brought her to the medical college hospital and admitted there for few months. She had taken tablet Escitalopram 10 mg HS and tablet Clonazepam 0.5 mg HS and had continued the same treatment till the last month. As the symptoms improved, she stopped the medication without any consultation so relapse of current episode occurred.

History of Past Medical-Surgical Illness

She has no history of fever/trauma/headache/vomiting/confusion/disorientation/memory disturbances/neuropathy/head injury/meningitis/encephalitis/epilepsy/delirium/typhoid/TB/syphilis.

Family History

Genogram (in three generation)

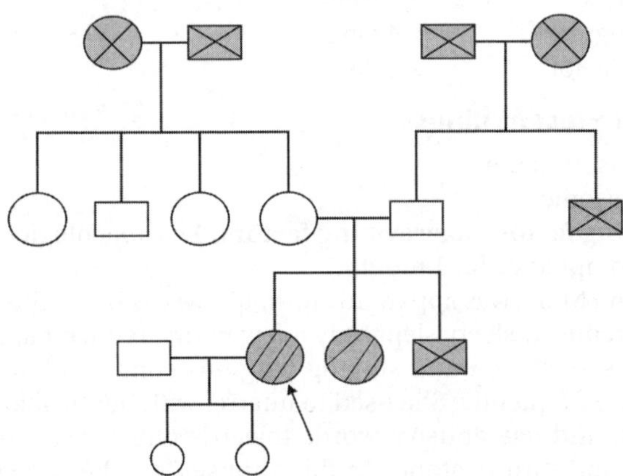

Details of Family Functioning

She belongs to a middle class nuclear family. No consanguinity between parents.

History of Illness in the Family

History of suicide for her paternal brother and has history of Bipolar Mood Disorder (BPMD) for her younger sister. No history of delinquency, personality problems, substance abuse, epilepsy, mental retardation, any hereditary medical illnesses.

Personal History

Birth and Early Development

- **Antenatal period:** Uneventful. Mother's health was adequate during this period. No history of pregnancy induced hypertension/ bleeding/infections, radiation exposure or use of teratogenic drugs.
- **Intranatal period:** Full term normal institutional delivery. Baby cried soon after birth. No birth defects.
- **Postnatal period**: No history of Postnatal complications such as cyanosis/convulsions/jaundice and postpartum psychosis for mother.

Childhood History

- **Infancy**: Developmental milestones (motor, adaptive, developmental, social) are normal for the age.
- **Behavior and emotional problems**: No history of sleep disturbances/thumb-sucking/nail-biting/temper tantrums/bedwetting/ stammering/tics/mannerisms/attention deficits/impulsivity/disobedience/fears/worrying/lack of self-confidence/attention seeking behaviors.
- **Emotional problems during adolescence:** No history of running away from home/delinquency/smoking/drug taking/truancy/any other.

Educational History

She started going to school at the age of 5. She had poor academic performance and studied upto 10th standard. No disciplinary problem but had adjustment problem with friends and so changed the school 3 times. She maintained good relationship with teachers. She was interested in group play.

Occupational History

Unemployed

Menstrual History

- She achieved menarche at the age of 14.
- She had regular cycles and duration of flow was 5 days.
- No physical and psychological symptoms to current cycle.
- Last Menstrual Period.

Sexual History

- Secondary sexual characters appeared at the age of 14.
- She had anxiety related to puberty changes. She had average level of knowledge regarding sex.
- No history of sexual abuse/premarital/extramarital sexual relations.

Marital History

She had arranged marriage at the age of 20. Her husband was 30 years old at the time of marriage. She had satisfactory sexual and interpersonal relationship with her spouse.

Obstetrical History

She has two children. No abnormalities associated with pregnancy and puerperium.

Premorbid Personality

- Interpersonal relationships: Extrovert
- Attitude to self: Thought to others
- Attitude to others: Positive
- Attitude to work and responsibility: Has decision making power, acceptance of responsibility, flexibility
- Use of leisure time: Sedentary
- Predominant mood: Optimistic
- Reaction to stressful events: Poor frustration tolerance
- Religious belief and moral attitudes: Adequate
- Habits
  - Eating pattern: Follows mixed diet
  - Elimination: Normal
  - Sleep: Adequate
  - No use of drug, tobacco, alcohol, other psychoactive substances.

MENTAL STATUS EXAMINATION

Date:
Time:

General Appearance

- Appearance: Looks same as that of stated age

- Body built: Ectomorphic
- Hygiene and grooming: Well groomed
- Mode of entry: Came willingly
- Posture: Normal
- Gait: Steady
- Facial expression: Happy
- Eye to eye contact: Maintained
- Gesture: Exaggerated
- Rapport: Spontaneously established
- Attitude towards the examiner: Cooperative
- Hallucinatory behaviors: Absent
- **Psychomotor Activity:** Increased
- **Other disorders**- restlessness and agitation.

Speech

Speech sample of client.
Nurse: Tell me about your home.
Patient: 'I have two children and grand daughters. My husband always says that the children are not his own. He used to say that my daughter is like crow. But I replied that crow has also had beauty (then singing song)...crow crow....... I used to sing this song for my grand daughters. They are very cute like me and I take care of them very well. They are studying in my own school. I feel happy...singing song.
Initiation: Spontaneous
Reaction time: Shortened
Rate: Rapid
Amount/productivity: Increased
Tone (loudness): Increased
Prosody of speech: Maintained
Relevance: Sometimes off target
Stream: Tangential
Coherence: Flight of ideas
Others: Pressure of speech present

Thought

Form: Flight of ideas
Stream: Tangentiality
Content: Delusions
Nurse: Do you think that others are trying to kill/harm you?
Patient: Yes my relatives brought me to this place for taking my properties as I have so many properties...
Inference: No delusion of persecution present.

Nurse: Do you have any special powers?
Patient: Yes I am Devi. I can able to know everything surrounding the world.
Inference: No delusion of grandiosity present.
Nurse: Do you think that others are noticing you/tell about you?
Patient: No
Inference: No delusion of reference.
Nurse: If anyone trying to influence you?
Patient: No
Inference: No delusion of control absent.
Questions are asked to elicit other delusions but are absent.

Depressive Ideations

Nurse: Do you have any hope for your future?
Patient: Yes
Nurse: Do you think that nobody is going to help you?
Patient: No
Nurse: Do you think that you have no worth?
Patient: No
Nurse: Do you want to harm yourself?
Patient: No.
Inference: No ideas of hopelessness/helplessness/worthlessness/suicidal ideations.
Nurse: Do you have any irrational fears?
Patient: No
Inference: No phobia

Possession

Nurse: Do you feel that somebody is putting thoughts in your mind?
Patient: No
Inference: No thought insertion.
Nurse: Do you feel that your thoughts are taken away by somebody?
Patient: No
Inference: No thought withdrawal
Nurse: Do you feel that your thoughts are broadcasted in TV or in other medias?
Patient: No
Inference: No thought broadcasting
Nurse: Is there any thought repeatedly came into your mind
Patient: No
Inference: No obsession

Emotion

Mood

Nurse: How are you/how do you feel now?
Patient: I am happy
Subjective: Happy
Objective: Elated mood
Affect-appropriate and congruent

Perception

Hallucinations
Nurse: Do you hear any voice that others are unable to hear?
Patient: No
Inference: No auditory hallucination
Nurse: Do you see anything which are not seen by others?
Patient: No
Inference: No visual hallucination
Nurse: Do you have any strange smells?
Patient: No
Inference: No olfactory hallucination
Questions asked to elicit other hallucination but are absent.
No Illusion.

Cognitive Functions

Consciousness: Conscious
Orientation
Time
Nurse: What is the time now?
Patient: Morning
Place
Nurse: Which is this place?
Patient: Medical college
Person
Nurse: Who is taking care of you in the hospital?
Patient: Husband
Inference: Oriented to time, place and person
Memory
Immediate
Nurse: Can you recall name of 3 objects after 5 minute: pen, mobile, car?
Patient: Pen, car, mobile
Recent
Nurse: Where were you yesterday?
Patient: Medical college

Remote

Nurse: Can you say your date of birth?
Patient: 1969 (Verify with relatives)
Inference: Immediate, recent and remote memory intact.
Attention:

	Nurse	Patient
Digit forward test:	1 - 4	1–4
	2 - 5 - 8	2–8
	9 - 2 - 5 - 1	5–2–1
	6 - 2 - 8 - 3 - 7	2–3–5
	Nurse	Patient
Digit backward test:	4 - 1	1–4
	8 - 5 - 2	2–5=8
	1 - 5 - 2 - 1	1–2–1
	7 - 3 - 8 - 2 - 6	2–6

Inference: Attention not aroused normally.

Concentration

Tests: Serial subtraction
Nurse: Subtract 7 from 100 and say 5 digits backward
Patient: 93, 85..I do not know [75 sec]
Nurse: Subtract 3 from 40 and say 5 digits backward
Patient: 37.. [15 sec]
Nurse: Subtract 1 from 20 and say 5 digits backward
Patient: 19,18,17, singing song ...[30 sec]
Inference: Concentration is not sustained.

Intelligence

General Fund of Information

Nurse: Can you name four districts in Kerala?
Patient: Thiruvananthapuram, Kottayam, Kollam, Alappuzha, Ernakulam.
Nurse: Which is our national animal?
Patient: Tiger
Inference: Adequate general fund of information.

Arithmetic Ability

Listen to the following problems and answer:
Nurse: 2 + 4 = ?
Patient: 6
Nurse: 8–2= ?
Patient: 6
Nurse: 6 × 3= ?
Patient: I do not know
Nurse: 8/2 = ?

Patient: (no answer)
Nurse: Suppose you have bought two pens for 20 rupees and given a 50 rupees note. How much is the balance you have to get back?
Patient: 30 Rupees
Inference: She has average arithmetic ability.

Abstract thinking

Proverb test

Nurse: Can you say one proverb?
Patient: I do not know
Nurse: Can you tell the meaning of the following proverb?
'All that glitters is not gold'
Patient: I have so many gold. My gold is pure gold not glittering.

Similarity and Dissimilarity

Nurse: Can you say the similarity and dissimilarity of apple and orange?
Patient: Apple is red, orange is orange in color. Both are used for eating. I like apple.
Inference: She has poor abstract thinking in proverb test, but abstract level of thinking present in similarity, dissimilarity test.

Judgment

Personal

Nurse: What is your future plan?
Patient: Look after my daughters.

Social

Patient has over sociability and interacted with everyone in the ward.

Test

Letter Test
Nurse: What will you do when you saw a letter/an envelope with address?
Patient: I will take the letter and read it.
Inference: She has intact personal and social judgment, but impaired test judgment.

Insight

Nurse: Why are you admitted in this hospital?
Patient: I have no problem. My husband and relatives brought me to here.
Inference: Grade I insight.

SUMMARY

Mrs X 48 years has history of episodic psychiatric illness since 2016. She had the complaints of decreased sleep, decreased appetite, over religiosity, increased speech and violent behavior which is precipitated by drug noncompliance. Her paternal uncle and elder sister both have psychiatric illness. She is premorbidly extroverted but has poor frustration tolerance. On MSE, she is well groomed, hygienic and cooperative throughout the interview. She has increased psychomotor activity and irritable sometimes. She has pressure of speech, tangentiality, flight of ideas, mood congruent delusions such as delusion of persecution and delusion of grandiosity. She has impaired attention, concentration and social and test judgment and has grade I insight.

Provisional diagnosis: Bipolar Mood Disorder (BPMD) Current episode Mania with Psychotic features.

Model Question Paper

(Previous Question Papers of Kerala Nurses and Midwives Council)

SET 1

Max Marks: 75
Time: 3 Hours

1. Define the following: **(5 × 1 = 5)**
1. Perseveration
2. Delusion
3. Delirium
4. Euphoria
5. Mental retardation

2. Differentiate between the following: **(5 × 2 = 10)**
1. Suppression – Repression
2. Insomnia – Hypersomnia
3. Ego – Superego
4. Illusion – Hallucination
5. Agoraphobia – Acrophobia

3. Fill in the blanks: **(5 × 1 = 5)**
1. Permanent loss of intellectual efficiency is termed as ___________
2. The word schizophrenia meaning is ___________
3. Eating disorder with irresistible craving for food is ___________
4. Method of sexual arousal by exposure of one's own genitalia is ___________
5. Repetition of words or phrases of the examiner is ___________

4. Match the following: **(5 × 1 = 5)**

a. Alzheimer's disease – Projection
b. Anhedonia – Dementia
c. Waxy flexibility – Absence of speech
d. Defense mechanism – Catatonic schizophrenia
e. Mutism – Depression

5. **Enlist the following:** **(5 × 2 = 10)**
   1. Four techniques of supportive psychotherapy
   2. Four personality disorders
   3. Four types of delusions
   4. Four signs of parkinsonism
   5. Four important techniques of therapeutic communication.

6. **Write short notes on (any five):** **(5 × 4 = 20)**
   1. Nursing care of patient with withdrawn behavior
   2. Rights of mentally ill patients
   3. Principles of milieu therapy
   4. Obsessive compulsive neurosis
   5. Characteristics of a mentally healthy person
   6. Mental status examination.

7. **Give reasons:** **(3 × 2 = 6)**
   1. Suicidal threat of a person should not be ignored
   2. In postpartum psychosis the infant is separated from the mother
   3. The extremities of the patient is supported during ECT.

8. **Essay:** **(1 + 3 + 3 + 7 = 14)**
   1. Mr X 35-year-old is admitted in psychiatric ward with the diagnosis of schizophrenia
      a. Define schizophrenia
      b. List down the signs and symptoms of schizophrenia
      c. Briefly describe the medical management
      d. Write down the nursing care of a patient with paranoid schizophrenia.

   OR

   2. Mr Y 30 years is admitted in the ward with depression **(2 + 4 + 8 = 14)**
      a. Define depression
      b. What is the difference between psychotic and neurotic depression?
      c. Describe briefly the medical and nursing management of patients with depression.

SET 2

Max Marks: 75
Time: 3 Hours

1. **Define the following:** **(5 × 1 = 5)**
   a. Euphoria
   b. Psychiatric nursing
   c. Mutism
   d. Dementia
   e. Narcolepsy.

2. **Fill in the blanks:** **(5 × 1 = 5)**
   a. Fear of closed space is termed as ___________
   b. New word created by patient is ___________
   c. Complete absence of speech is ___________
   d. Moderate elevation of mood is ___________
   e. The awareness of oneself in relation to time, place and person is ___________.

3. **Match the following:** **(5 × 1 = 5)**
   a. Apathy – Habitual involuntary movement
   b. Sodium Valproate – Walking during sleeping
   c. Chlorpromazine – Mood stabilizer
   d. Mannerisms – Absence of affect
   e. Somnambulism – Antipsychotic

4. **Differentiate between the following:** **(5 × 2 = 10)**
   1. Illusion – Hallucination
   2. Transference – Counter Transference
   3. Repression – Regression
   4. Delusion of Persecution – Delusion of Self Accusation
   5. Echolalia – Echopraxia.

5. **Give reasons:** **(5 × 1 = 5)**
   a. Injection atropine is administered before ECT
   b. Lithium is contraindicated in pregnancy
   c. Antipsychotics are administered as deep IM injections
   d. Over discussions on delusions should be avoided
   e. Injection phenergan is administered alongwith injection serenace.

6. **List down the following:** **(5 × 2 = 10)**
   a. Four causes of mental illness
   b. Four phases of therapeutic nurse patient relationship
   c. Four types of personality

d. Four techniques of interview in psychiatric patients
e. Four legal issues in psychiatry.

7. Write short notes on (any five): **(5 × 4 = 20)**

a. Nursing management of client during ECT treatment
b. Psychiatric emergencies
c. Principles of psychiatric nursing
d. Misconceptions about mental illness
e. Milieu therapy
f. Mental retardation.

8. Essay: **(1 + 4 + 3 + 7 = 15)**

a. Define schizophrenia
b. List the types of schizophrenia
c. Explain the signs and symptoms of schizophrenia
d. Explain the nursing management of a patient with schizophrenia.

SET-3

Max Marks: 75
Time: 3 Hours

1. Define the following: **(5 × 1 = 5)**
   a. Illusion
   b. Mental status examination
   c. Regression
   d. Perseveration
   e. Community mental health nursing

2. Fill in the blanks: **(5 × 1 = 5)**
   a. Excessive day time sleeping by an individual is termed as ___________
   b. Fear of pain is ___________
   c. Writing or pictorial art to arouse sexual passion of the reader or viewer is ___________
   d. Intentional touching of another without the consent of the client is ___________
   e. The initial disturbance that results from stressful event is

3. Match the following: **(5 × 1 = 5)**

a. Serenace	–	Antiparkinsonian
b. Imipramine	–	Anxiolytic
c. Lithium	–	Antipsychotic
d. Lorazepam	–	Anticonvulsant
e. Eptoin	–	Antidepressant

4. Differentiate between the following: **(5 × 2 = 10)**

a. Obsession	–	Compulsion
b. Transference	–	Counter transference
c. Conversion reaction	–	Dissociative reaction
d. Precipitating cause	–	Predisposing cause
e. Individual psychotherapy	–	Group Psychotherapy

5. Give reasons: **(2 × 2 = 4)**
   a. Blood pressure should be monitored in patients taking antipsychotics
   b. Careful observation is necessary for patients with acute depression.

6. Enlist the following: **(5 × 2 = 10)**
   a. Four types of schizophrenia
   b. Four types of delusions
   c. Four phases of therapeutic relationships

d. Four community facilities
e. Four side effects of antipsychotics

7. Write short notes on (any five): (5 × 5 = 25)

a. Milieu Therapy
b. Nursing management of a client before and after ECT
c. Anxiety neurosis
d. Causes of mental illness
e. Prevention of suicide
f. Mental retardation

8. Essay: (1 + 2 + 8 = 11)

a. Define dementia
b. List down the types of dementia
c. Write down the nursing management of client admitted with senile dementia.

OR

a. What is depression
b. Enlist the cause of depression
c. Write the nursing management of a client with endogenous depression. (1 + 2 + 8 = 11)

SET-4

Max Marks: 75
Time: 3 Hours

1. Define the following: **(6 × 1 = 6)**
   a. Mental status examination
   b. Psychotherapy
   c. Dyslexia
   d. Anhedonia
   e. Dementia
   f. Judgment

2. Fill in the blanks: **(5 × 2 = 10)**
   a. Standard method of measuring level of consciousness is ___________
   b. Fear of open place is called ___________
   c. ___________ is the awareness about oneself
   d. ___________ is the persistent involvement of an adult in sex with children.
   e. Episode of binge eating followed by self condemnation is ___________

3. Match the following: **(5 × 1 = 5)**

a. Lithium	–	Akathisia
b. ECT	–	Phobia
c. Extra pyramidal symptom	–	Flat affect
d. Therapeutic community	–	Mood stabilizer
e. Apathy	–	Lucino Bini

4. Differentiate between the following: **(5 × 2 = 10)**

a. Repression	–	Compensation
b. Dementia	–	Delirium
c. Echolalia	–	Echopraxia
d. Obsession	–	Compulsion
e. Illusion	–	Hallucination

5. List down the following: **(5 × 2 = 10)**
   a. Four neurotransmitters
   b. Four methods of assessments in psychiatry
   c. Four component of therapeutic communication
   d. Four sexual deviations
   e. Four eating disorders

6. Write short notes on (any five): **(4 × 5 = 20)**

a. Principles of psychiatric nursing
b. Nursing management of patients with dementia
c. Prevention of suicide
d. Rights of psychiatric patient
e. Role of nurse in community mental health.

7. Essay: **(1 + 2 + 2 + 9 = 14)**

a. Define schizophrenia
b. What are the cause of schizophrenia
c. List down the signs and symptoms of paranoid schizophrenia
d. Explain the nursing management of a patient with paranoid schizophrenia.

Index

Page numbers followed by *f* refer to figure and *t* refer to table, respectively.

B

D

E

I

N

O

P

Q

R

S

W

Y

Z